IRON
YOGA®

IRON YOGA

Combine Yoga and Strength Training for Weight Loss and Total Body Fitness

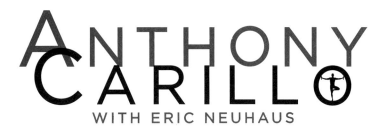

ANTHONY CARILLO

with ERIC NEUHAUS

RODALE

Photographs by Darryl Estrine
Photographs on page xii and xiii courtesy of Action Sports International

Book design by Susan P. Eugster

Library of Congress Cataloging-in-Publication Data

Carillo, Anthony.
    Iron yoga : combine yoga and strength training for weight loss and total body fitness / Anthony Carillo with Eric Neuhaus.
        p.   cm.
    Includes index.
    ISBN-13 978–1–59486–209–0 paperback
    ISBN-10 1–59486–209–5 paperback
    1. Aṣṭāṅga yoga.   2. Weight training.   3. Physical fitness.   4. Weight loss.   I. Neuhaus, Eric. II. Title.
RA781.68.C37   2005
613.7'046—dc22   2005005636

Distributed to the trade by Holtzbrinck Publishers

6   8   10   9   7   5   paperback

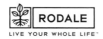

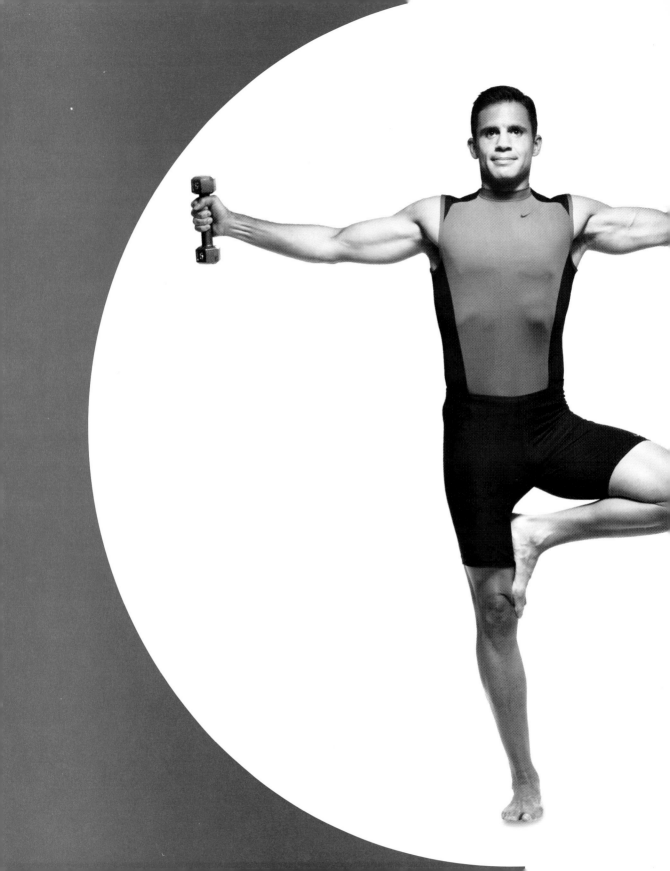

CONTENTS

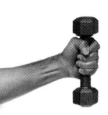

ACKNOWLEDGMENTS

I would like to express my sincere gratitude to the following individuals who either played a huge role in this project, in some way were a part of the creation of Iron Yoga, or at some point influenced and touched my life in so many positive ways.

Mom, you have lived each day of your adult life with the desire to be the most incredible mother three boys could possibly have—we are so fortunate. Dad, ever since I was a little boy, you have always been my role model and hero. By example, you taught the meaning of respect, trust, hard work, and loyalty. From storytelling, help with homework, cheers at many baseball games, marathons, and ironman races, to encouraging us to reach for the stars—you both were always there for us. Thank you for your love, guidance, and devotion, and for instilling a solid foundation of values and morals that are my pillars of strength and endurance.

My brothers, John and Joey—you guys are not only amazing brothers, but best friends. Your integrity, honesty, dedication to family, and tremendous hearts and souls make me proud to be your older brother. Thank you for your support and encouragement and for always being there.

My aunts, uncles, cousins, and late grandparents, thank you for making Sunday my favorite day of the week when I was growing up. The memories I have of family vacations and holidays together will last a lifetime.

My mother- and father-in-law, sisters-in-law, Marina, Laura, Stacey, and Christine, thank you for opening your arms and welcoming me into your family.

My nephews, Thomas and Christopher, and nieces, Daniela and Holly, you all bring tremendous joy to my life, and it's terrific being your uncle.

The team of professionals at Rodale—Margot Schupf, Andrew Gelman, Susan Eugster, Christine Bucks, Patricia Field, Jessica Roth, Sara Sellar, Nicole Lewis, Jessica Guff, Donald Silvey, and Bob Mezan. Also thanks to Peter Demas and Penny Price. Thank you for giving me the opportunity to create this book and video and share my workout with others. You all have made this experience such a positive one.

Eric Neuhaus, my coauthor, thanks for your assistance with my manuscript and your expertise and creativity in turning my workout and story into a book. We once talked about how it was so important for you to master the synergy between the mind-body-spirit and mind-muscle connections—you have definitely done so. Thanks for your patience and hard work.

Laleli Lopez, without your help and interest, all of this would not have been possible. You first planted the seed that the media should be alerted to my Iron Yoga creation, and you were instrumental in making the appropriate connections. Your countless hours, enthusiasm, and drive are greatly appreciated.

A special thanks to Maryann Donner, group fitness director of New York Health & Racquet Club, for giving me the opportunity to teach my first Iron Yoga class in Manhattan and taking such an interest in my growth and development. Thank you also to the following group fitness directors for including Iron Yoga on their schedules: Jill Oppenheimer, Michelle Ruocco, and Kim Mayer of Equinox; Dorian Pascoe and Paul Weiss of Asphalt Green; Jo-Ann Houston of the New York Athletic Club; Sharon Abeelhamid of Sharon's Underground/Verol's Gym; and John Boyd of Chelsea Piers. Thank you also to Jay Travis, director of marketing at New York Health & Racquet Club, for getting Iron Yoga exposure on TV, in magazines, and in newspapers.

My Uncle Dudy for creating the Iron Yoga logo, layout of my Web site, and the sketch of this book's cover design. Your artistic talent is extraordinary, and I will always cherish the hours of stories you have shared with me spanning a remarkable 48 years of working on Madison Avenue as an art director.

Darryl Estrine and your staff for an incredible photo shoot of the Iron Yoga workout.

Lori Roth and NIKE for providing the apparel and yoga mats for our photo shoot.

Drew Hong for constructing the www.ironyoga.com Web site.

Van Cushny, Ronald Kaye, and Anne Vranos for your counseling, business, and legal advice.

Swim Coach Doug Stern for the opportunity to teach Iron Yoga during your triathlon camp on the beautiful beaches of Curaçao at sunset.

Alan Ley and Andre Lapar of the USA Triathlon Coach Education and Development Center for giving me the opportunity to present an Iron Yoga workshop to newly certified triathlon coaches.

Maryann Herklotz for the opportunity to present an Iron Yoga workshop to the physical and occupational therapists at Memorial Sloan-Kettering Hospital.

My cousin and schoolteacher Louisa Markewitz for inviting me to Tangier Smith Elementary School to present Iron Yoga to the first- and second-grade students.

Nancy Lazar for the opportunity to teach Iron Yoga to your employees at International Strategy & Investment Group, Inc.

My friends David Lipsius, Tim Doran, Bob Gordon, Andrew Motola, David Schneider, Swim Coach Steve Shtab, teammates at Runners Edge and Asphalt Green Tri Club. It has been so incredibly fun taking my ironman journey with you and sharing training and racing experiences. Thank you also David Lipsius for your insight and advice relating to Iron Yoga and the numerous brainstorming sessions we shared.

My friends Andrea Rhodes and Amy McKoy, you were my first Iron Yoga students. Thank you for the hours you let me practice teaching and experimenting with new sequences and weight-training exercises. Your positive feedback and praise gave me the confidence that I could teach this workout to others.

My friend Judi Delmaestro for inviting me to watch the 1992 NYC Marathon. Feeling the energy of thousands of runners along First Avenue was the motivation and incentive for me to race the following year and eventually led to my love of long-distance running.

All of my Iron Yoga students and clients who have practiced with me over the past 2 years. It has been extremely rewarding and fulfilling for me to present you this challenging workout and watch you grow and improve and achieve your health and fitness goals.

Finally, I'd like to thank my wife, Amy. You radiate and glow with such incredible energy. Thank you for sharing your experiences in the fitness world and helping me to become a better instructor. I am so fortunate to share my life with you—you make my dreams become reality and my passions feel so fulfilling and rewarding.

FROM IRONMAN TO IRON YOGA

The starting gun fired, and I sprinted into Popolopen Lake to begin the swim of my first triathlon: the West Point Sprint in upstate New York. Surrounding me were hundreds of swimmers all jockeying for the lead—kicking, elbowing, and punching me as they passed me by. Almost immediately, I went into oxygen debt and started gasping for air. My arms and legs became so heavy that I no longer had strength to stroke and kick, and less than 100 yards later, I went into survival mode. I began to tread water and let my competitors swim ahead, but 3 minutes later, the next wave of swimmers started to beat me up and attack all over again.

Panic set in while tears filled my eyes. And for those few moments, I had no desire to ever race a triathlon again. But 25 minutes later, I finally exited the water with such relief and then had to find the energy to get on my bike and begin cycling.

The race leaders had come out of the water well below 15 minutes, so I was very far back and had a lot of catching up to do on the bike and run. This part of the race soon became fun. On the bike, I was now flying past many of the triathletes who had kicked, punched, and swum over me in the water. I had a somewhat respectable finish for my first triathlon after a much stronger bike and run. Crossing the finish line brought a tremendous feeling of satisfaction, fulfillment, and accomplishment. I knew I was in this sport for the long haul. Since that sprint triathlon in the summer of 1997, I have gone on to finish 13 ironman triathlons, including the past five Super Bowls of triathlons—the Hawaii Ironman World Championship.

By now, you're probably wondering what the connection is between the ironman and yoga. As with yoga, there is an ironman mystique that is extremely powerful in forging the connection between mind and body. If you're not familiar with it, the ironman is one of the most grueling races in the world, which includes a 2.4-mile swim, a 112-mile bike ride, and a 26.2-mile run. This race distance challenges you not only physically but mentally and spiritually as well. The finish time limit is 17 hours, and I can definitely attest to the fact that some serious soul-searching takes place over the course of this long day.

I started thinking about yoga one day after watching a yoga workout show on TV—a show where two lively instructors from a popular New York yoga studio taught yoga on a beautiful beach in sunny Jamaica. The first time I watched the show, I recall an incredible feeling of calmness and relaxation—though the life of a triathlete typically is anything but calm and relaxed. It's always a challenge to fit in a workout, waking up before the sun rises to bike or run in darkness while stressing over family commitments and career responsibilities.

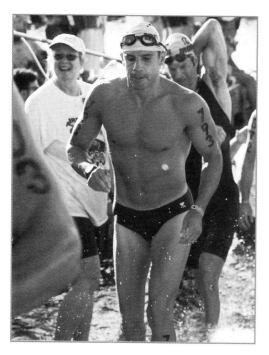 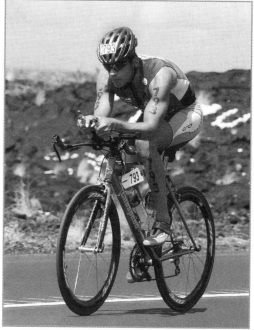

So, I incorporated yoga into my triathlon training program in December 2000, practicing four or five sessions per week. As a certified public accountant in private industry, it was often difficult for me to get to a yoga class due to the time constraints of a full-time job and training for triathlons—upward of 25 hours per week. The majority of my yoga practice was done in my living room—either watching a video or going through my own series of favorite poses.

When I first started yoga, it was very difficult for me to learn to breathe the proper "yogic" way. As with many athletes, my breath had always been very short and shallow, coming from just the chest and rib cage. I also found that due to the tremendous tightness of my hamstrings, hip flexors, and lower back muscles from all of my cycling and running, many of the yoga poses were just simply uncomfortable.

The one-legged balancing poses were completely frustrating. I could never hold the pose and balance for more than 2 breaths before toppling over. Nonetheless, I was determined—the instructors made everything look so incredibly easy, and they were in such great shape.

Scenes from the Hawaii Ironman Triathlon World Championship, 2004, culminating with my wife, Amy, who was cheering me on from the sidelines, running hand-in-hand for the last 50 yards.

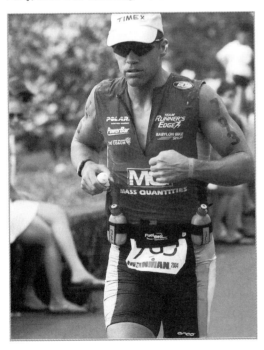
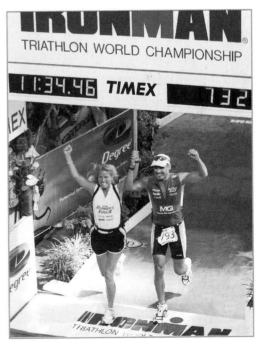

FROM IRONMAN TO IRON YOGA

I figured my weaknesses—breath, inflexibility, and balance—would tremendously improve my abilities in triathlon if I could somehow turn them into strengths.

Consequently, I arranged my training schedule so I would wake up at 5 a.m., go for my morning swim, bike, or run, and then return home to practice 30 minutes of yoga before I left for work. My yoga workout soon became an obsession—equally as important as any swimming, biking, or running session. If, on a given day, I had an opportunity to perform only one workout, I often chose yoga. I found that yoga was such a positive complement to my multisport activities.

I was certainly feeling stronger. My improved flexibility enhanced my range of motion. I became more streamlined and balanced in the water, my running stride length increased, and my cycling power improved. I opened up a whole new energy source by incorporating a proper manner of breathing. At the same time, I sharpened my focus and concentration skills, which are so important during training and competition. Most important, yoga was keeping me healthy and injury-free and accelerating my recovery time from intense workouts and races.

A week after racing at the 2002 Ironman USA triathlon in Lake Placid, New York, I was practicing yoga in my living room one afternoon and performing my favorite standing pose, Warrior 2 (see page 95). I could feel my leg muscles start to burn the deeper I got into this challenging lunge pose. As I stared at myself in a mirror, I wondered how I could get that same muscle burn for my upper body—my shoulders and arms. They didn't seem to be working as intensely as my legs.

In the corner of the room, I had a stability ball and a pair of 5-pound dumbbells. (Along with my yoga practice, twice a week I performed a series of upper-body weight-training exercises with dumbbells while balancing on the stability ball.) I picked up both dumbbells and returned to the Warrior 2 pose. With my arms extended straight out to the sides and now holding an additional 5 pounds each, my arms and shoulders definitely felt just as pumped as my lower body. I looked in the mirror and noticed something interesting about my arms. They were holding the dumbbells in a perfect position to perform a weight-training exercise.

Over the next 90 minutes, I combined common weight-training exercises with my favorite yoga poses. This was the beginning of what I now call "Iron Yoga." The "Iron" refers not only to the dumbbells but to my passion for the ironman triathlon. During the past 2 years, I have perfected the workout while teaching Iron Yoga classes at health clubs in New York City and Long Island.

Now that you've read about how I developed Iron Yoga, it's time for you to take the next step and experience the power of Iron Yoga for yourself. You will be amazed by the synergy you'll feel between yoga's mind-body-spirit connection and weight training's mind-muscle connection. Iron Yoga is a truly unique training workout that can help you achieve your health, fitness, and weight management goals.

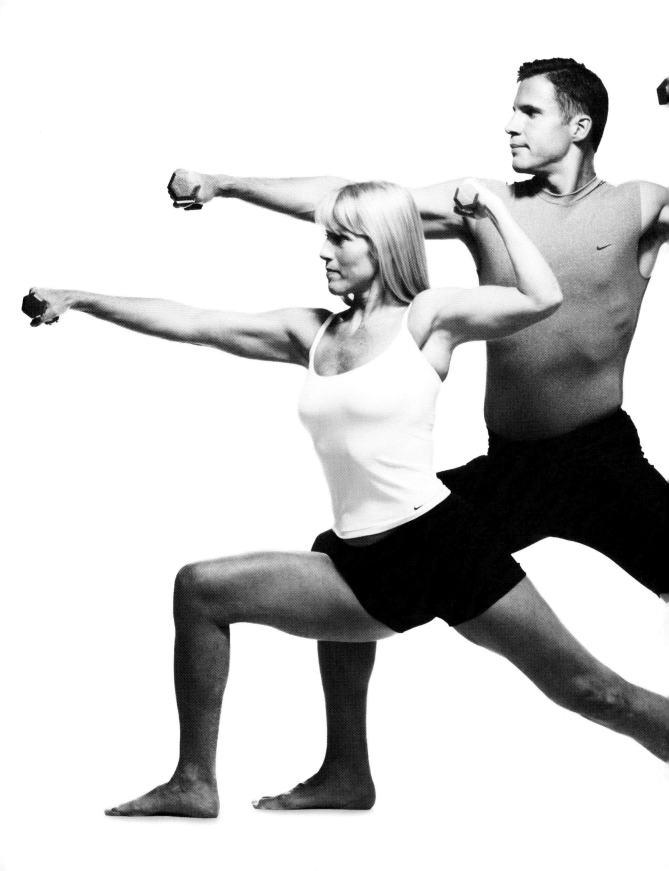

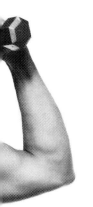

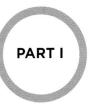

PART I

UNDERSTANDING
IRON YOGA

The Buddha once said, "The mind is everything; what you think, you become." As you begin to understand the concepts and philosophy of Iron Yoga, never underestimate the power of your mind. Indeed, you will find that Iron Yoga challenges the physical limits of your body, but never lose sight of the fact that those limits are, by and large, constructed in your mind. So for the time being, set aside any of these limitations and allow your mind the limitless capacity to understand this new experience called Iron Yoga.

CHAPTER 1

WHAT IS IRON YOGA?

Yoga is such an incredible discipline for the mind, body, and spirit. It's no wonder the ancient ritual has been practiced all over the world for more than 5,000 years and is more popular in the United States today than ever before. Virtually anyone can practice yoga. Whether you are looking to lose a few pounds and tone your body; delay the aging process and expand longevity; recover from an ailment, disorder, or injury; train the mind and body for sport and competition; or just live the yoga lifestyle, incorporating the practice of yoga into your life can be tremendously rewarding and beneficial to your overall health and well-being.

There are many different styles of yoga. The most traditional forms are called Hatha. Hatha yoga originated in ancient India and represents the physical aspect of yoga. Through a series of poses involving physical strength and stamina as well as breathing exercises, Hatha yoga was developed as a means to meditation.

Over the years, Hatha yoga has been modified to reflect the teachings of a particular organization or teacher. You've probably heard of yoga classes called *Ashtanga, Iyengar, Viniyoga, Kundalini, Kripalu, Bikram,* and *Power Yoga.* These are all styles of Hatha yoga, each emphasizing different breathing techniques and a different physicality. Some styles can be very physically demanding, while others are more meditative and contemplative.

Ashtanga yoga is known for its fast-paced movements in which postures flow from one to another (this flow is called vinyasa). Iyengar yoga involves precise alignment and symmetry. Viniyoga uses the breath along with movement and is slower paced. Kundalini's purpose is to awaken the "serpent power" within us through breath control, chanting, and meditation. In Kripalu yoga, three stages of postures lead to a spontaneous meditation in motion. Bikram yoga is a sequence of 26 poses held for up to 10 seconds, practiced in a room heated between 80° and 105°F.

Finally, one of the newest and most popular styles is called Power Yoga. Power Yoga combines traditional Hatha yoga poses with fluid movements and deep-breathing techniques to create a high-energy workout. Although Power Yoga moves faster than Viniyoga, it does incorporate meditation and breathing along with movement and encourages students to listen to their bodies. Over the past few years, the many styles and variations of yoga have expanded into the entire fitness field. No longer is yoga confined to special schools and exclusive spas—you can now find yoga classes in just about every gym, health club, and recreation center across the country.

Yoga's popularity as a form of fitness and physical exercise has allowed me to add this new dimension of combining weight-training exercises using light dumbbells with Power Yoga poses.

With Power Yoga as the foundation, the essence of Iron Yoga is the beautiful synergy between weight training and yoga. Weight training is a discipline that requires a connection between mind and muscle, while yoga is an art form that connects mind, body, and spirit. When the two are combined in my Iron Yoga practice, you benefit physically, mentally, and spiritually.

When you are working out in the gym or at home with machines or free weights for the upper body—say chest or back, shoulders or arms—you are generally targeting one specific muscle group at a time. Iron Yoga is an incredibly intense, challenging, full-body workout because when you are balancing on one leg, for example, you are performing a series of exercises for your upper body like some of the ones you may be familiar with: Shoulder Overhead Press, Triceps Kickback, and Chest Flye. What's so unique about Iron Yoga is that while you are in a Power Yoga pose, your legs are active, your abdominal region is engaged, and every weight-training movement is controlled by breath and performed with continuous tension through a full range of motion. In the next chapter, you'll learn more about these principles and techniques for practicing Iron Yoga.

BENEFITS OF IRON YOGA

What makes Iron Yoga distinctive is that it has the combined benefits of yoga and weight training all in one workout. Iron Yoga will help you . . .

Improve lean muscle mass. Increased lean muscle helps fire up your metabolism and assist with losing weight. The more lean muscle mass you have, the easier it will be to control and maintain your weight. Muscle acts like a fat-burning machine. When you're losing weight, the goal is to replace fat with lean muscle. Performing a variety of weight-training exercises with low-weight resistance executed in a slow and controlled manner is a great way to stimulate lean muscle.

Increase your flexibility and range of motion. When your body is tight and stiff, you are more likely to get injured. This applies to playing your favorite sport or performing everyday activities like carrying groceries and pushing the baby stroller. Iron Yoga helps you keep your muscles and joints limber and active.

Sharpen your mental focus and concentration skills. The Iron Yoga practice increases oxygen and bloodflow to the brain. It helps keep your mind focused no matter what you're doing—whether you're running a marathon or working on a business proposal. A focused mind can better handle the rigors of everyday life.

Develop proper breathing techniques. One of the best ways to reduce stress and tension is through deep breathing. When you consider that by some estimates, 80 percent of all illness is stress related, you'll probably find that practicing Iron Yoga can help keep you out of the doctor's office.

Enhance your functional strength and muscular endurance in your legs and core areas. Good posture is important to so many aspects of a healthy life. Whether you're sitting or standing, awareness of the muscles in your legs and core helps you keep your body in proper alignment. Muscular endurance and functional strength are also important to enhance any cardio activity such as running, cycling, swimming, skiing, and rowing.

Create balance and symmetry. Your body wants to naturally balance. This centering of your body and creating symmetry is so vital to your overall health and well-being. When your body is out of balance, it is often very common to feel fatigued or become ill or injured. If your mind is agitated or wandering, you'll probably end up swaying and wobbling. Iron Yoga helps to restore symmetry and rejuvenate your whole body.

IRON YOGA POSES

There are many types of yoga movements. Some movements, such as balancing poses, are more active and challenging. Others are more passive and meditative. The Iron Yoga practice incorporates four types of yoga poses:

STANDING POSES

These poses are the foundation of the Iron Yoga practice. Whether you are standing on two feet or balancing on one leg, standing poses help to center your body and your mind and help you feel grounded. The physical challenge of standing or balancing creates strength and stability for your lower body. Some examples of standing poses are Chair (see page 42), Tree (see page 51), Warrior 2 (see page 73) and Warrior 3 (see page 108), and Crescent Lunge (see page 78).

SEATED POSES

While standing poses challenge your body and mind, seated poses are more reflexive and meditative. Many of the seated poses in Iron Yoga require flexibility of the lower back and spine. Some examples are Seated Wide Angle Sequence (see page 159), Seated Forward Bend (see page 155), and Bound Angle (see page 156).

PRONE POSES

These are poses performed when you are facing the floor, either on your hands and knees or simply lying on your stomach. Prone poses are very good for strengthening your shoulders and back. These are very active and demanding poses. Some examples are Bird Dog/Flying Airplane (see page 137) and Locust (see page 144).

SUPINE POSES

These are poses performed when you are lying on your back. While prone poses activate and build strength, supine poses help you relax and release tension. Lying on the floor is a great way to feel alignment and symmetry. An example of a supine pose is Reclined Twist (see page 154).

IRON YOGA MOVEMENTS

The weight-training movements in Iron Yoga improve lean muscle mass and build strength in the upper body. The Iron Yoga practice incorporates two basic types of weight-training movements you should become familiar with:

ISOLATION MOVEMENTS

An isolation movement targets only one muscle group, such as your biceps or triceps. This is also called a single-joint movement because only one joint comes into play. For example, when working your biceps and triceps, the joint in play is your elbow. Isolation movements are great for sculpting and toning a specific muscle. Two good examples of isolation movements are the Concentration Curl (see page 76) and Triceps Kickback (see page 109).

COMPOUND MOVEMENTS

A compound movement combines two or more joints and targets large or primary muscle groups. Some fitness experts consider compound movements more efficient than isolation movements because you work several muscles at once. The Chest Press (see page 55) and Lat Pulldown (see page 54) are good examples of compound movements because they target the large muscles of your chest and back respectively and involve two joints—elbow and shoulder.

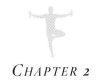

CHAPTER 2

PRINCIPLES OF IRON YOGA

Now that you know what makes Iron Yoga unique, it's time to deepen your understanding of the Iron Yoga practice. The foundation of the Iron Yoga practice are four basic principles. I call these principles "The Four Connections" because they all involve some form of mental or physical connection. Whether it's mind to breath or breath to body, the focus is on completely integrating your mind, breath, and body while practicing Iron Yoga. Some of these principles are easy to grasp, and others are more subtle. Take the time to read through each principle carefully, then do the "Try This" exercise. These simple exercises will help you put the principles into practice so that, in Part II, you can more readily apply them to the Iron Yoga workout.

PRINCIPLE #1: CONNECT MIND WITH BREATH

As with other forms of yoga, the most basic principle of Iron Yoga is the breath. Therefore, it's important to understand how to breathe properly. Sure, we all breathe as an unconscious part of living. It's a necessity of life. But Iron Yoga requires a special type of breathing called *ujjayi*.

Ujjayi breathing initiates from the abdominal region and diaphragm. You inhale through your nose, keeping your mouth closed, and feel your belly expand at the start of each breath. You fill up your lungs and feel your rib cage and chest expand. Then, you exhale through your nose, keeping your mouth closed, feeling the contraction of your chest and rib cage, and squeeze out the last bit of air by contracting your abdominal region. It's important to feel and hear your breath. You should feel your breath deep in the back of your throat and make the sound of the letter "h" (as in *hahhh*) by gently constricting your throat's opening. You know you have it right when your ujjayi breath sounds like the breathing of Darth Vader in the movie *Star Wars*. Each complete ujjayi breath should take 4 or 5 seconds for an inhale and 4 or 5 seconds for an exhale.

(My students sometimes tell me that they have trouble breathing exclusively through the nose. Due to congestion or allergies, you may sometimes have difficulty breathing through your nose. First, don't stress about it. That's counterproductive to yoga. Try inhaling through your nose and exhaling through your mouth. If that's not possible at all, then simply breathe in and out through your mouth.)

TRY THIS: UJJAYI BREATHING EXERCISE

Lie comfortably on the mat facing up with your body completely relaxed and your eyes softly closed. Focus on taking deep, long, full breaths through your nose while keeping your mouth closed. Try to develop a timing of your breath, making your inhalations and exhalations even, steady, and consistent. It sometimes helps to count each inhalation and exhalation in seconds—1 one thousand, 2 one thousand, 3 one thousand—to establish a steady breathing rhythm.

Next, place your hands gently over your belly. Start to inhale, and feel with your hands your belly rise and expand. Now exhale, and feel with your hands your belly lower and contract. Perform 5 breaths with your hands over your belly and then 5 breaths with your hands removed.

Do this same exercise with your hands first under your rib cage and then on top of your chest. Notice the same rising and expanding on an inhalation and the same lowering and contracting on an exhalation. Again, perform 5 breaths with your hands in place and 5 breaths with your hands removed.

You'll notice the relaxing effect on your mind and body when you have successfully tuned into your breath. This is ujjayi breathing—which is so energizing, calming, cleansing, and healing to your body. It is impossible to practice Iron Yoga and derive the benefits without first making this connection of mind with breath.

PRINCIPLE #2:
CONNECT MIND-BREATH WITH MUSCLE

Like the roots and trunk of a tree, your legs and core are your foundation. Whatever pose you are in and whatever weight-training exercise you are performing, you need to keep your legs active and your core engaged. You can't simply let your lower body relax and go along for the ride. There needs to be a mind-muscle connection with your legs and core. It will amaze you how intense a muscle burn you will feel in your legs, glutes, abs, and obliques. I'll tell you more about connecting your mind and *engaging* other muscles and parts of your upper body in the next chapter. For now, let's focus on your legs and core.

TRY THIS: LEGS ACTIVE EXERCISE

Stand tall with your feet together and your legs straight. Place your hands gently on the front of each thigh. Notice how your front thigh muscles, your quadriceps, are soft and relaxed. Now, lift both kneecaps without fully locking out. Your quadriceps will automatically begin to contract, becoming firm and *active*. Next, place your hands gently on the back of each thigh. These are your hamstring muscles. Again, lift your kneecaps and feel these muscles become active. Finally, place your hands over your buttocks. This strong muscle group is the gluteal region, or glutes. Lift the cheeks of your buttocks and feel the glutes contract and become active.

TRY THIS: CORE ENGAGE EXERCISE

In the same standing position, place your hands over your belly. Contract your abs by drawing your navel up and in toward your spine. This is what it feels like to have your *core engaged*.

PRINCIPLE #3:
CONNECT MIND-BREATH-MUSCLE WITH MOVEMENT

In Iron Yoga, the ujjayi breath controls all movement of the upper and lower body. When you are flowing from one yoga pose to the next, you are always breathing deeply with steady inhalations and exhalations. The inhalation will create positive energy flow and rejuvenate your mind and body. The exhalation will release negative energy flow and relax your mind and body. In Iron Yoga, you will also be connecting your breath with all of the weight-training exercises. The movement of your arms and the dumbbells is always synchronized with the inhalation and exhalation.

Let's start with some weight-training basics. A single movement of a weight-training exercise with the dumbbells is called a *repetition*. A repetition can be divided into two parts. When you lift the dumbbell going against gravity, that's called the *concentric* or *positive* phase of the movement. When you lower the dumbbell going with gravity, that's called the *eccentric* or *negative* phase of the movement. Throughout the positive and negative phases of the movement, you must keep *continuous tension*. Continuous tension relates to maintaining pressure or tension on the muscle without allowing it to rest or relax through its fullest range of motion. You may find it a little difficult to keep the tension when you're lowering the dumbbell since you've got gravity on your side. This is when your mind-muscle connection must be stronger and more disciplined.

The breathing pattern in Iron Yoga is different than the one you might be familiar with in your regular weight-training program. Normally, when you are working out with weights, the simple rule is weight up, exhale; weight down, inhale. In other words, you exhale on the *exertion* phase (lifting the weight up) and inhale on the *rest* phase (lowering the weight down). In Iron Yoga, however, there never is a *rest*. You keep continuous tension through the entire range of motion while working a muscle both concentrically and eccentrically.

When practicing Iron Yoga the first few times, the breathing and movement pattern may be confusing. That's why it's important to follow the breathing cues precisely as instructed in the next section. You'll see that each step of the practice has an inhalation and exhalation direction. If you've been practicing other forms of yoga, then the breathing flow will come to you very naturally. If you're new to yoga, it will take some time to coordinate the breath with the movement.

Why is all this important? It all comes back to the breath. The slower, deeper, and fuller the breath, the slower the movement. The slower the movement, the more continuous the tension and the stronger the muscle contraction. The stronger the muscle contraction, the greater shaping, toning, and sculpting for the body.

TRY THIS: MOVEMENT WITH BREATH EXERCISE

Stand tall with your feet together and your legs straight. Grip a 3- or 5-pound dumbbell in your right hand. Relax your right arm by your right side and rotate your right hand so your palm is facing forward. Place your left fingertips gently on the front of your right upper arm. Notice how your upper arm muscles—your biceps—are soft and relaxed. Squeeze the dumbbell tightly in your hand and immediately feel your biceps become firm and tense. That's the feeling you're looking for—you've just *engaged* your biceps. Your entire right arm, from your wrist to your shoulder, is now *active* and prepared for the movement of a weight-training exercise.

The next goal is to synchronize your movement with your breath. Keep your left fingertips on the right biceps muscle, so you can feel the work of the muscle. Inhale and begin to curl the right dumbbell up to your right shoulder. Maintain *continuous tension* through the full range of motion as you contract the biceps more intensely. Make sure to time the movement with the length of your inhalation—the slower the breath, the slower the movement. When the inhale breath stops, the movement stops. The dumbbell should now be at shoulder height, and your biceps at a point of *peak contraction*. Again, this part of the repetition is called the *concentric* or *positive* phase.

Now, begin your exhale breath and start lowering the dumbbell. Maintain continuous tension through the same full range of motion and keep your biceps *active*. Time the movement with the length of your exhalation—the slower the breath, the slower the movement. When the exhale breath stops, the movement stops, and the dumbbell should be at the start position. Again, this part of the repetition is called the *eccentric* or *negative* phase.

It is important to keep the durations of your inhale breath and exhale breath even. It is crucial to never *hold* your breath. Every weight-training exercise is performed in this controlled manner, whether you are targeting your arms, shoulders, chest, or back. The connection of mind-breath-muscle with movement will eliminate the possibility of cheating and reduce your chance of injury.

PRINCIPLE #4:
CONNECT MIND-BREATH-MUSCLE
WITH STATIC CONTRACTION

In Principle #3, I explained how you should synchronize each complete breath (inhalation and exhalation) with the movement of the repetition. After you complete 2 repetitions (and 2 complete breaths), you perform the last repetition using a special technique called *static contraction*.

A static contraction is actually an advanced bodybuilding and weight-training technique.

It is a powerful way to make the connection between your mind and muscle. It challenges your mind and body, but the ultimate result is that you are enhancing the peak contraction of the muscle. Simply put, a static contraction means pushing or contracting your muscle against resistance and then holding that contraction for a few seconds. That hold is what's called the *static contraction*.

Here's how it works in the Iron Yoga practice. On your inhalation (of breath 3), you lift the dumbbell as you did before. Now, instead of exhaling and lowering the dumbbell, you hold it in the peak contraction position. As you hold this position, you squeeze and contract the muscle tighter and stronger. You should feel an intense muscle burn and pump, even with light dumbbells. At the same time, you continue to breathe. This is the hardest part. You're not holding your breath but rather breathing to *enhance* the peak contraction and intensify the mind-muscle connection. You exhale (to complete breath 3) while still holding the same position, and then inhale again (to start breath 4) while still holding the same position.

During these breaths at static contraction, it's important to remember to keep your inhalation and exhalation deep, long, and full. Try to create strength and energy throughout your body while you inhale, and calmness and relaxation throughout your body while you exhale. Learning to correctly perform this static contraction technique takes incredible concentration and discipline. It's challenging to both the mind and body.

TRY THIS: STATIC CONTRACTION EXERCISE

Stand tall with your feet together and grip a dumbbell in your right hand. Activate your legs and engage your core. As before, place your left fingertips gently on your right biceps, so you can feel the work of the muscle during the exercise.

Breath 1: Engage your right biceps. Inhale and curl the right dumbbell to your right shoulder. Exhale and lower the right dumbbell to the start position. Keep continuous tension through the full range of motion.

Breath 2: Repeat as above.

This is the static contraction:

Breath 3: Engage your right biceps. Inhale and repeat as above. Hold at peak contraction. Exhale, hold the movement, and enhance the peak contraction.

Breath 4: Inhale, hold the movement, and enhance the peak contraction. Exhale and lower the dumbbell to the start position.

PUTTING IT ALL TOGETHER

As you begin your Iron Yoga practice, keep all of these principles in mind. You will see that they are the nuts and bolts of Iron Yoga. Remember, it all comes back to your breath. So ask yourself throughout the practice, *am I breathing?* This may sound simple, but as you begin to focus on the poses and getting your body into proper alignment, it's easy to let your breath fall to the wayside. Take a few minutes at the beginning of your practice to review these principles. You may even want to do the practice exercises in this chapter for the next few weeks as your mind-breath-body becomes accustomed to the Iron Yoga fundamentals.

With consistent practice, these principles will become second nature. The challenge of the Iron Yoga workout has no limitations. As your lower body, core, and ujjayi breath get stronger, you will be able to go deeper and longer into each pose. As your upper body gets stronger, you can increase the weight of the dumbbells or increase the number of repetitions for a movement. (Make sure to never increase the dumbbell weight if it will cause you to sacrifice form or risk injury.) You can also increase the number of breaths you perform during a static contraction.

GETTING STARTED WITH IRON YOGA

With the principles of Iron Yoga under your belt, you're almost ready to get started. In this chapter, I'll give you the basics to get your practice off the ground. In the meantime, as you begin to prepare for your Iron Yoga practice, think about your goals. What do you hope to achieve from your Iron Yoga practice? Do you want to lose weight? Do you want to find a way to decompress after a stressful day at the office? Do you want to become stronger and leaner? Do you simply want to become more physically fit? After you're clear about your expectations for practicing, write down your goals. This will help you find the time and keep you motivated to practice Iron Yoga for years to come.

WHEN TO PRACTICE

There's no best time to practice Iron Yoga. Above all, you need to find a time that works for you. Whatever time you choose to practice, make sure you allow ample time for your body to digest food—90 minutes after a snack or 2 hours after a heavier meal. If you practice first thing in the morning, you'll already have an empty stomach that won't interfere with your workout.

Ideally, Iron Yoga should be practiced two or three times a week. That initial goal will help you develop familiarity with the unique Iron Yoga sequences. If you're new to yoga, then it will take some time to really learn the poses. If you've been practicing other types of yoga, then you'll probably catch on to the technique a little faster.

Keep in mind that no matter how often you practice Iron Yoga, it's not meant to take the place of your regular fitness program or yoga practice. I find that Iron Yoga works best when you supplement it with activities you already do. In fact, many of my students say that Iron Yoga has actually helped them in their other yoga classes. Iron Yoga is also a great way to improve your performance in other fitness activities such as running and cycling. (Remember when I told you how it was a great benefit to my triathlon training?) That's why, in Iron Yoga for Sports (see page 167), I've outlined ways that Iron Yoga can help remedy some problems in popular sport and fitness activities.

WHAT YOU NEED (EQUIPMENT)

One of the great things about Iron Yoga is that you don't need a lot of expensive fitness equipment, gizmos, or gadgets. Just about everything listed here you can find in your local sporting goods store. What's more, you don't need a lot of space to practice Iron Yoga—an office, small studio apartment, or basement can work perfectly.

Yoga mat: A mat will help keep your body from sliding on the floor. Even if you practice on carpeting, I suggest you purchase a mat. Some carpeting can be just as slippery as a smooth floor.

Dumbbells: Iron Yoga is not about lifting heavy weight. When you're first starting out, I suggest a pair of dumbbells each weighing 2 or 3 pounds. After you feel comfortable with the movements, you can increase the weight to 4 or 5 pounds. The emphasis is not on the amount of dumbbell weight, but on the power of your mind-muscle connection.

Mirror: For those new to yoga, I suggest practicing in front of a mirror. Alignment and posture are very important in yoga. This will give you a chance to see if your body is in the correct position. Seeing yourself in a mirror will also assist you in the balancing poses and with proper form of weight-training exercises.

Clothing: You should wear clothing that is light, comfortable, and breathable so that your body feels unrestricted when moving.

Bare feet: You should practice Iron Yoga, like all forms of yoga, with bare feet. In order to get the proper traction in the standing and balancing poses, you need to be able to hold steady without slipping. Wearing socks will cause you to slide around.

A quiet space: As much as possible, choose a room or area that's quiet and free from interruptions. A ringing phone or loud television can distract you from the concentration you'll need for the practice.

PRACTICING SAFELY

The most fundamental rule of Iron Yoga—and any type of yoga for that matter—is to *listen to your body*. Never take a pose to a level that will risk injury to your body. The deepness of a pose will be controlled with proper yogic breathing and should go only to a point that your body can accept. A pose should never bring pain and discomfort to any part of the body. The Iron Yoga workout stresses perfect posture and alignment, precise execution of form with every weight-training exercise, and controlled movement flows from one pose to another. Learn to recognize the difference between *muscle burn* caused by deepening a pose or intensifying the peak contraction and *pain* to the knees, ankles, feet, hips, back, shoulders, or elbows caused by incorrect execution of a pose or weight-training exercise. Muscle burn is good—and it's this feeling that will lead to positive results in shaping, toning, and sculpting the body. Joint pain is bad and must be avoided and prevented during every practice.

MODIFICATIONS

Every pose in Iron Yoga can be modified depending on your level of experience in practice and your own physical limitations. I've listed some modifications in the instructions for the specific movements. You'll see those later on. In short, the easiest modification when you're doing a weight-training movement is to simply put the dumbbells on the floor and perform the movement without any weight at all.

If you have a specific circumstance that may limit your practice, take special note of the modifications for the following situations.

Back pain. Generally, back pain is caused by poor posture. Many of us sit for long periods of the day typing at computers or staring at computer screens. Weak abdominals combined with tight hamstrings can also be a cause. Believe it or not, tension is also a major cause of neck and back pain. The meditative and relaxing aspect of Iron Yoga can greatly help you release tension, particularly in those problem areas.

The Iron Yoga practice can help by strengthening your abs and lower back muscles. The floor poses in Chapter 7, such as Bow and Cow/Cat, are great for stretching your lower back and neck.

Hamstring stretches such as Standing Forward Bend (in Chapter 6) will also be helpful. Boat and Locust (in Chapter 7) will help strengthen your lower back.

Modifications: You should make sure to bend your knees during the forward fold and stretching movements. Remember to perform each pose gently, and if you feel any strain to your lower back or neck, stop immediately.

Pregnancy. During pregnancy, you need to exercise extreme caution about practicing Iron Yoga. As you would for any exercise program during pregnancy, consult your doctor. If you have never practiced Iron Yoga, I suggest you wait until after you give birth to start. If you've been practicing Iron Yoga prior to your pregnancy, then I recommend you stop during your first trimester—and make sure you limit the intensity and length of the practice when you resume during your second and third trimesters. Some of the benefits of Iron Yoga to you and your baby are that it relaxes your whole body and relieves back problems.

Modifications: You should avoid deep forward bends, spinal twists, and any pose that puts pressure on your uterus. In fact, you should avoid lying on your stomach altogether. You should move slowly and gently and avoid any jumps or quick movements, because your joints will naturally become looser during pregnancy due to increased levels of certain hormones. Be careful not to overstretch your muscles because this could lead to serious injury.

Seniors. Iron Yoga can be very beneficial for seniors. One of the most significant benefits of Iron Yoga is the deep abdominal breathing and focus on the breath. Deep abdominal breathing expands the chest and improves the respiratory system. The strength movements with light weights in Iron Yoga can help maintain strong bones and prevent bone loss (osteoporosis), particularly for women. Bone loss for women can actually start much earlier—in your thirties—so it's really never too early to begin Iron Yoga. For seniors, good balance and stability are particularly important in helping to prevent falls. The balancing poses such as Tree and Eagle in Chapter 6 are perfect for developing those skills.

Modifications: For balancing poses, you should use a chair, or stand against the wall for additional support.

KNOW YOUR BODY

One of the most important aspects of the Iron Yoga practice is to connect your mind with not only your breath but with a specific muscle. When I describe how you should perform each of the movements, I ask you to "engage" a specific muscle or group of muscles. In other words, you should make a mental connection with the muscle before you start to work it. This is a very powerful technique and one used by many bodybuilders.

To help connect your mind with your muscles, it's important that you understand some basic anatomy. Most of you probably know these basic body parts, but even so, take the time here to learn the names and locations of the muscles, because I will be referring to them quite a bit throughout the rest of the book.

ABS, RIGHT AND LEFT OBLIQUES (Rectus Abdominis, Transverse Abdominis, Internal Obliques, External Obliques)

This is a group of muscles that make up your core region. These muscles help cinch your waist as well as stabilize and protect your spine. The obliques help with movements such as rotating and side bending as well as movements against gravity such as sitting up, jumping, and climbing. Boat (see page 148), Half Moon (see page 105), Oblique Crunch (see page 150), and Oblique Twist (see page 80) specifically target the core area.

LATS (Latissimus Dorsi)

The lats are the largest muscles of your back. They extend all the way from your pelvis to your shoulder blades by wrapping around the ribs. The Lat Pulldown (see page 54), Lat Pullback (see page 56), and Row (see page 44) weight-training exercises really help to build these muscles.

TRAPS (Trapezius)

The traps are large, triangular muscles that extend from the base of your skull to about two-thirds of the way down your back. These muscle help you raise your shoulders and extend and stabilize your head. They also keep your shoulders squared off. The Shoulder Shrug (see page 38) and Upright Row (see page 39) weight-training exercises target this area.

PECS (Pectoralis)

This muscle group is located in the front of the chest and under the breasts. It flexes and rotates your arms when your hands are pressed together in front of your chest. It is impor-

(continued on page 24)

KNOW YOUR BODY

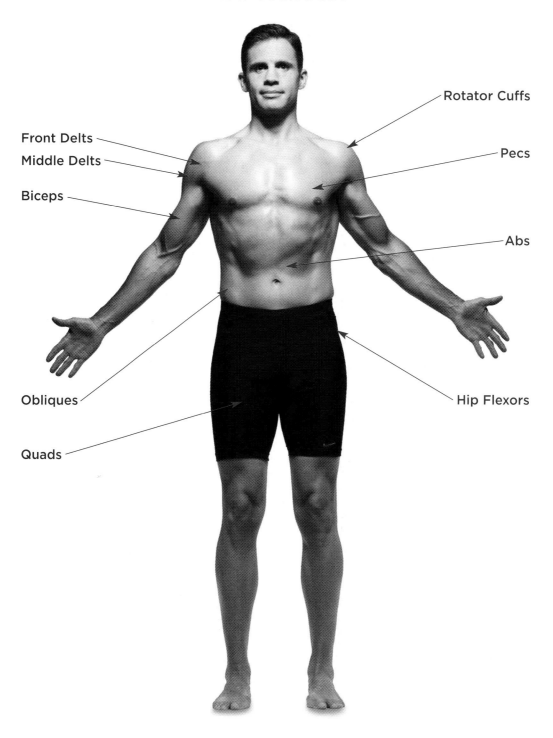

Rotator Cuffs

Front Delts

Middle Delts

Pecs

Biceps

Abs

Obliques

Hip Flexors

Quads

UNDERSTANDING IRON YOGA

KNOW YOUR BODY

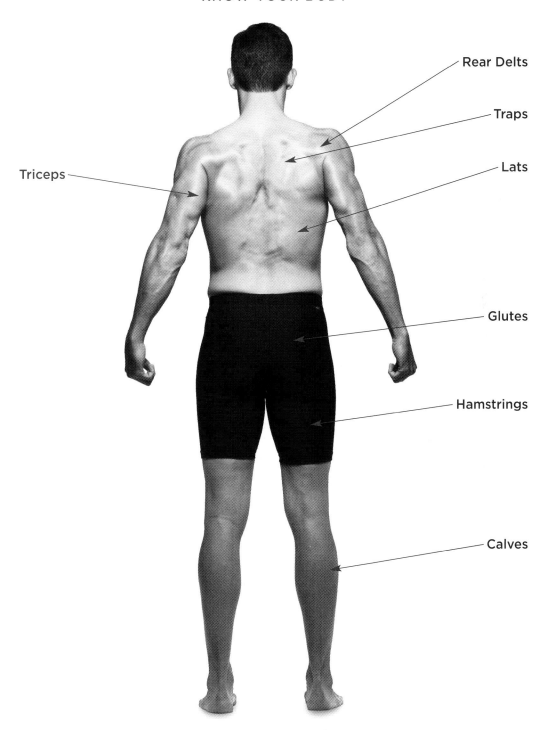

Rear Delts

Traps

Triceps

Lats

Glutes

Hamstrings

Calves

tant to strengthen these muscles to help steady your shoulders. You'll find the Chest Press (see page 55) and Chest Flye (see page 57) weight-training exercises particularly helpful for toning and shaping your pecs. The poses in the Sun Salutation (see page 81), Plank and Chaturanga (see page 84) are also great for working the chest.

DELTS (Deltoids)

The delts make up your shoulders and consist of three muscles: anterior or front, medial or middle, and posterior or rear muscles. The delts help you rotate your arms inward and outward. The delts also help raise your arms to the front, side, and rear of your body. The following exercises will strengthen your delts: Front Raise (see page 64), Lateral Raise (see page 74), Rear Lateral Raise (see page 43), Reverse Flye (see page 58), Shoulder Overhead Press (see page 53), and Modified Lateral Raise (see page 127).

ROTATOR CUFFS

This is a group of muscles closely surrounding your shoulder area. The rotator cuff helps stabilize and rotate your shoulder joint. The External/Internal Rotation (see page 67) movements help to target and strengthen this muscle group.

BICEPS

The biceps are made of two heads—a short and a long—that extend from the top of your shoulder joint all the way to your elbow and forearm. Strong biceps help you flex your shoulder and forearm. You use these muscles in the various curl movements such as Biceps Curl (see page 74), High-Arm Hammer Curl (see page 41), and Concentration Curl (see page 76).

TRICEPS

The triceps are made up of three heads that extend from your shoulder to your elbow on the back of your arm. These muscles support the elbow joint when you're extending and pushing. When you strengthen your triceps, you help give the back of your arm a more toned and sculpted appearance. All of these exercises are great for your triceps: Triceps Pressdown (see page 66), Triceps Kickback (see page 109), and Triceps Overhead Extension (see page 126).

HIP FLEXORS

The hip flexor is the point where the thigh bone meets the pelvis. You can feel the hip bone on either side of your pelvis. The muscles here include the major and minor psoas, which work together to lift your leg in front of your body. Generally, these muscles become tight from sitting. Pigeon pose (see page 141) is a great stretch for your hip flexors.

GLUTES (Gluteus Maximus)

The glutes are responsible for the rounded shape of your butt. They are a very thick and powerful group of muscles that help you walk, stand up, climb, and sit. They also help control the movement of your hips. The Power Lunge Sequence (see page 69), Bird Dog/Flying Airplane (see page 137), and Eagle (see page 111) will create a good muscle burn for your glutes.

QUADS (Quadriceps)

The quads are some of the strongest muscles in your body. They are comprised of four smaller muscles extending from your hips to your knees in the front of each thigh. The quads help extend the leg and bend the knee. Since your quads also help stabilize the knee, strengthening your quads can help you prevent injury to your knee. The Leg Extension (see page 110) and Power Lunge Sequence (see page 69) are particularly good for developing your quads.

HAMSTRINGS (Biceps Femoris)

While the quads comprise the muscles in the front of your thigh, the hamstring muscles are a group of three muscles running down the back of your thigh. The hamstring extends from the hip joint to the knee. When it's flexed, this muscle helps you bend the knee joint, extend the thigh, and rotate your leg out to the side. The Power Lunge Sequence (see page 69) and Warrior 3 (see page 108) help to strengthen the hamstrings. The Leg Curl (see page 110) is also a great hamstring developer.

CALVES (Gastrocnemius)

The calf is a large rounded muscle at the back of your lower leg. The calf helps to keep the ankle and foot stabilized as well as aligned and moving properly. Downward-Facing Dog (see page 85) is a great stretch to help keep this muscle supple, long, and flexible. The Calf Raise (see page 118) will also specifically target this area of the lower leg.

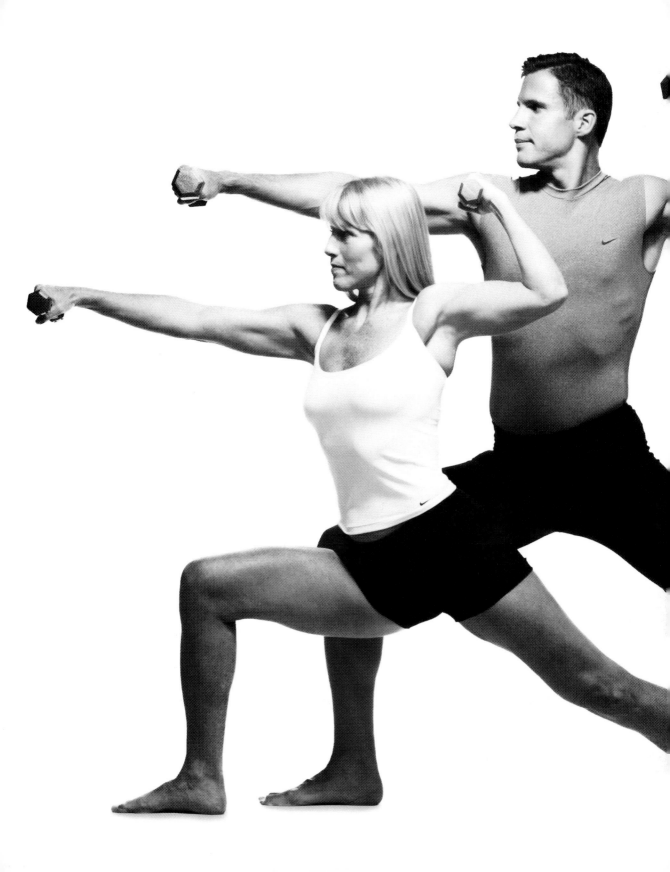

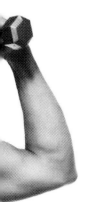

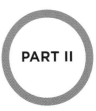

PRACTICING
IRON YOGA

Part II of this book is a step-by-step guide to your practice. While I've given you the principles and theory of Iron Yoga in Part I, Part II is about doing. With these powerful tools, you can now practice Iron Yoga on your own. I suggest reading through Part II a few times before actually beginning the workout so that you can become familiar with the language and flow of the movements. If you're new to yoga, this might take more time. If you've done yoga before, many of the poses will be familiar, but you'll need to focus on integrating the weight-training exercises.

CHAPTER 4

BEFORE YOU BEGIN

The complete Iron Yoga practice (Chapters 5 to 8) represents a 60-minute workout. I've divided the practice into chapters, with each chapter representing a component of the Iron Yoga practice.

Within each chapter, the poses are organized into sequences. The sequence of poses is called a *vinyasa*. In designing the sequences, I have combined poses that work both your upper and lower body. I have also included poses that counterbalance and are complementary to other poses. A counterbalancing pose is one that uses the muscles opposite those you just used. For instance, at the end of Single-Leg Balance Sequnce—Left Leg (see page 129), I have included an excellent quad stretch called Dancer's pose. This pose is designed to counterbalance and stretch the muscles you have been working up to that point.

In addition to the Iron Yoga movements, you'll also find some traditional yoga poses that do not utilize added resistance with dumbbells. These poses are excellent for increasing strength and improving flexibility. You'll also see that I've included two Sun Salutation Sequences (see pages 81 and 130). The Sun Salutations help to rejuvenate and energize the full body. They also give your body a break from the weight-training movements.

Pay careful attention to the breath as you proceed through each sequence. I have given you specific directions for when to inhale and when to exhale. Follow these directions closely to maintain the proper connection of breath with movement. Even though you're learning the poses for the first time, synchronize your movement to your breath as best you can. The more you practice, the easier this will become and the greater results you'll see and feel.

At first, you might not have the strength and stamina to complete the entire workout. Or some days, you might be short on time. That's okay. Do what feels right for you and work your way up to completing the entire practice. If you decide to shorten the program to your needs, always make sure you begin with the Warmup (see page 33). You should also make sure to work both the right and left sides of a sequence. For instance, if you decide to do the Tree Sequence—Right Leg (see page 47), make sure to balance your workout by completing the Tree Sequence—Left Leg (see page 60). The same holds true for the Power Lunge Sequences (see pages 69 and 91) and Single-Leg Balance Sequences (see pages 103 and 116). Always be sure to end with the Cooldown (see page 153), no matter what the length of your practice. The Cooldown is a time for relaxation and meditation. This is very important in yoga. The relaxation and meditation help you release any remaining tension and stress from your body.

Throughout the Iron Yoga program, you will find some key words to help guide you through the poses and movements:

Prepare. This is a preparatory pose that helps you focus your mind and connect with your breath. Generally, this will be a form of Mountain pose.

Transition. This is a movement that takes you from one yoga pose to the next.

Start position. This is the starting position of a weight-training movement.

Static contraction. This relates to Principle #4 (see page 13), in which you hold a weight-training movement through two breaths (breaths 3 and 4) of a repetition.

Now you are ready to begin. Here are some Iron Yoga tips to keep in mind as you embark on your Iron Yoga journey:

- Consult your doctor before starting Iron Yoga.

- Work within your own capabilities and limitations.

- Don't force a movement or stretch. If you're feeling tension, relax and breathe into the pose.

- Visualize the movement or pose you are going to do with specific focus on the muscles you are going to be working.

- Generally, pain is a signal that you've gone too far. Stop immediately.

- Don't hurry your movements. Move slowly into each pose.

- Let your eyes relax by softening your focus and turning your attention inward.

- Have fun! Enjoy challenging your mind and body.

Chapter 5

WARMUP SEQUENCE

The Iron Yoga Warmup Sequence is designed to awaken your muscles and prepare your body for the invigorating workout that follows. Most important, this sequence will help you connect with all the muscle groups of your body. Developing a steady breathing rhythm and synchronizing the movement with the breath are the essence of Iron Yoga.

The foundation pose for this warmup is one of the most basic yoga poses—Mountain pose. Mountain pose improves your posture and focus.

Chair pose, which you'll also be doing in this sequence, generates heat and warmth in your body. After 8 breaths in this pose, your legs will be screaming!

The biceps are one of the easiest muscle groups to feel and connect with, and that's why I've included the High-Arm Hammer Curl in this warmup. This exercise will be your first opportunity to perform a static contraction. Learn, understand, and feel what it's like to engage the muscle and create a peak contraction for the muscle with your breath and powerful mind-muscle connection.

You'll be returning to Mountain pose many times throughout the Iron Yoga practice. This strong standing pose will allow you to refocus and reconnect with the breath, especially after an intense pose or sequence of poses. If you get tired or need a break during the practice, you can simply return to Mountain pose.

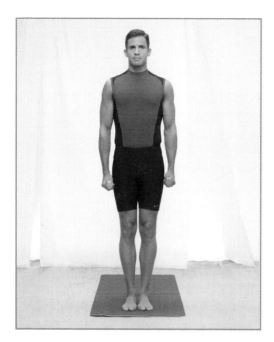

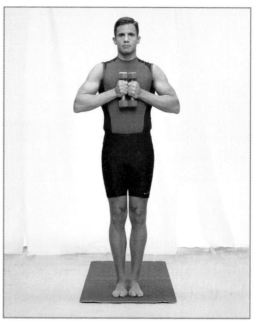

1. Mountain/Dumbbells at Sides

Stand at the front center of your yoga mat, holding one dumbbell in each hand, with your arms comfortably at your sides. Place your heels slightly apart and your big toes together. Spread wide the rest of your toes. Feel the four corners of your feet firmly press into the mat. Lift your kneecaps to activate your quads, hamstrings, and glutes. Draw your navel up and in toward your spine to engage your core. Release your shoulders down and back away from your ears. Keep your torso tall, your chest out, and your head neutral. Soften your face, and gaze at a point directly level with your eyes. Hold for 2 to 4 breaths.

2. Mountain/Dumbbells over Heart

Lift the dumbbells to your chest. Rotate your palms to face your body and gently press together both dumbbell heads over your heart. Softly close your eyes and begin to connect with your breath. Create a meditative state of mind and body. Use your breath to ease your mind and relax your body. Focus on the yogic style of ujjayi breathing. Remember to keep your mouth closed and breathe only through your nose. Initiate the breath from the abdominal region, feeling your belly, rib cage, and chest expand on your inhale and contract on your exhale. Establish an equal timing and rhythm of your inhalations and exhalations. Feel and hear your breath. On each exhale, press together stronger both dumbbell heads. Pressing together the dumbbells creates continuous tension and activates the muscles in your upper body. Begin to develop a mind-muscle connection for your upper body—shoulders, arms, chest, and back. Breathe in positive energy and exhale out all negative energy. Hold for 4 breaths. Softly open your eyes.

34

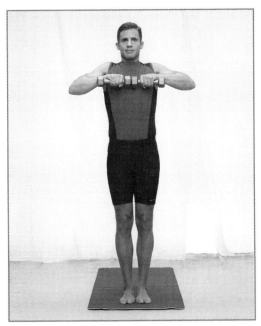

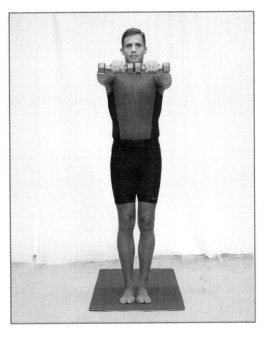

3. Start Position

Rotate your palms downward so just the top dumbbell heads are pressing together. The goal for each movement is to flow with your breath and maintain continuous tension through the full range of motion. Prepare to make a mind-muscle connection with every muscle group in your upper body. Remember to keep your legs active and your core engaged while performing all the upper-body weight-training exercises.

4. Chest Press

Engage your pecs, inhale, and press the dumbbells straight forward, keeping your arms at shoulder height while pressing together the top dumbbell heads.

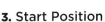

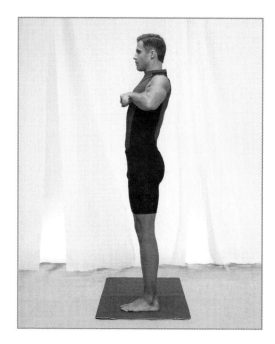

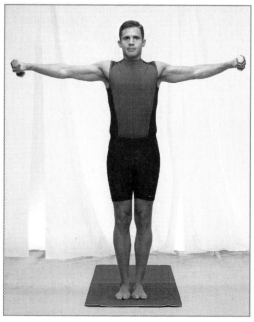

5. Lat Pullback

Engage your lats, exhale, and pull back the dumbbells to your chest, keeping your elbows up and out to the sides while pressing together the top dumbbell heads.

6. Triceps Kickside

Engage your triceps, inhale, and straighten your elbows, extending the dumbbells out to the sides. Keep your elbows at shoulder height.

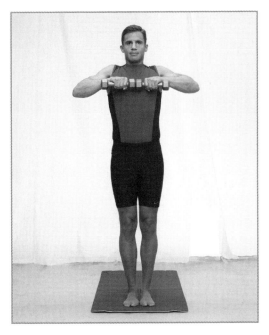

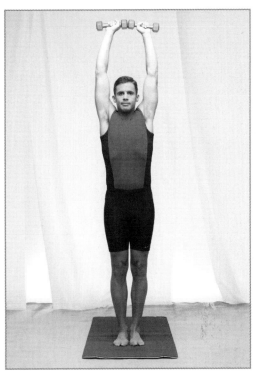

7. Biceps Curl

Engage your biceps, exhale, and bend your elbows, curling the dumbbells to your chest and pressing together the top dumbbell heads.

8. Shoulder Overhead Press

Engage your front and middle delts, inhale, and press the dumbbells straight overhead while pressing together the top dumbbell heads. Feel your biceps close to your ears at full extension.

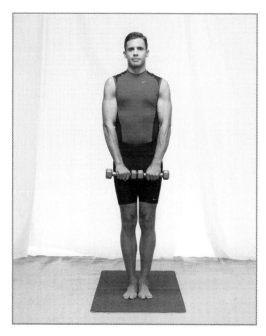

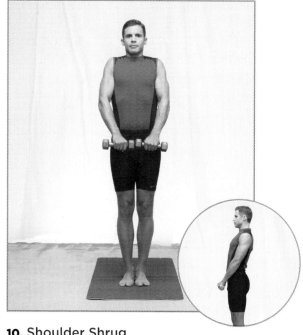

9. Straight-Arm Pulldown

Engage your lats and pecs, exhale, and pull down the dumbbells over the front of your head (think pulling over a barrel) and down to your thighs. Keep your arms straight through the full range of motion while pressing together the top dumbbell heads.

10. Shoulder Shrug

Engage your upper traps, inhale, and shrug your shoulders straight toward your ears and round them back (see inset). Exhale, round your shoulders forward, and lower them straight down. Keep your arms straight while pressing together the top dumbbell heads and don't bend your elbows when you shrug your shoulders. Rotating and rounding the shoulders at the top of the movement helps to release any tightness and tension from the neck, shoulders, and upper back.

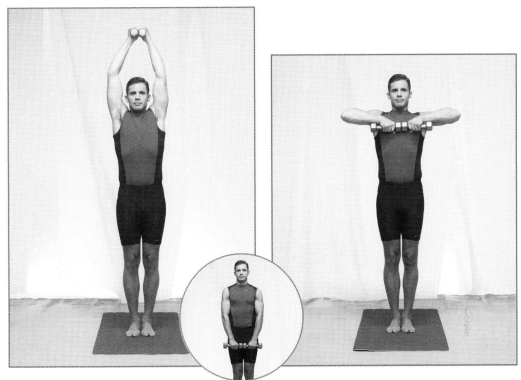

11. Full Overhead Lateral Raise

Engage your middle delts, inhale, and raise the dumbbells straight out to your sides, with your palms facing upward. Press together both dumbbell heads overhead, with your palms facing each other. Exhale and press the dumbbells down to your sides, with your palms facing downward, and press together the top dumbbell heads in front of your thighs (see inset). The downward movement should feel like you're pressing down water.

12. Upright Row

Engage your traps, inhale, and pull the dumbbells up the front centerline of your body to your chin while pressing together the top dumbbell heads. Spread your elbows wide, slightly higher than shoulder height. Try to lead the movement with your elbows and not pull with your hands.

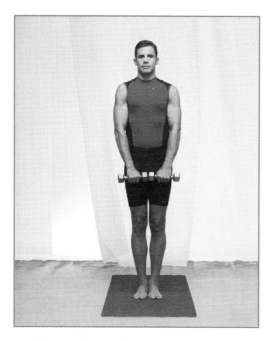

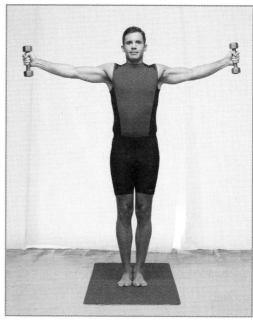

13. Triceps Pressdown

Engage your triceps, exhale, and press the dumbbells down the front centerline of your body to the fronts of your thighs while pressing together the top dumbbell heads.

14. Start Position

Inhale and raise the dumbbells straight out to your sides at shoulder height, with palms facing backward. Exhale and rotate your palms facing forward.

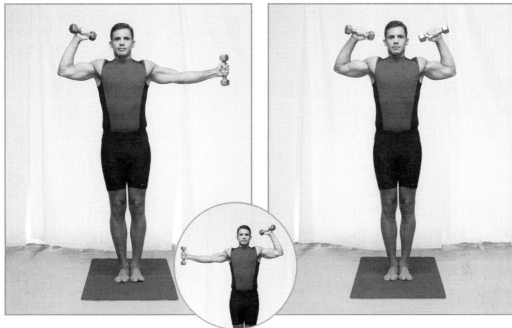

15. High-Arm Hammer Curl

Engage your right biceps, inhale, and curl the top right dumbbell head to your right shoulder. Exhale and press the dumbbell back to the start position (#14). Make sure to isolate the biceps rather than using the wrist and forearm when curling.

16. Repeat #15 with the left dumbbell (see inset).

17. Static Contraction

Inhale and repeat #15 with both dumbbells. Hold the movement at peak contraction. Exhale and then inhale to enhance the peak contraction. Exhale and press both dumbbells to the start position (#14).

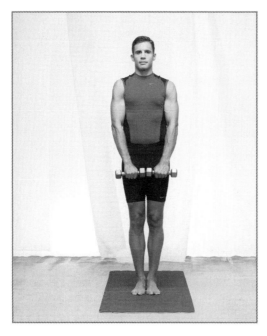

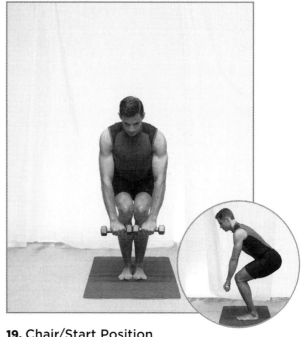

18. Transition

Stand in Mountain pose, pressing together the top dumbbell heads in front of your thighs.

19. Chair/Start Position

Inhale to prepare, exhale, and softly bend your knees. Lower the dumbbells in front of your shins while pressing together the top dumbbell heads. Shift your weight back by pressing firmly into your heels. Sit back into your buttocks and activate your glutes, quads, hamstrings, and calves. Your thighs should be almost parallel to the floor, and you should feel like you're sitting in a chair. Keep your torso at a 45° angle to the mat with your back flat. Release your shoulders down and back away from your ears, lift your chest, and keep your head neutral. You should not feel any strain in your neck. Maintain a straight line from your tailbone to the crown of your head (see inset). Gaze at a point on the floor about 2 feet in front of you.

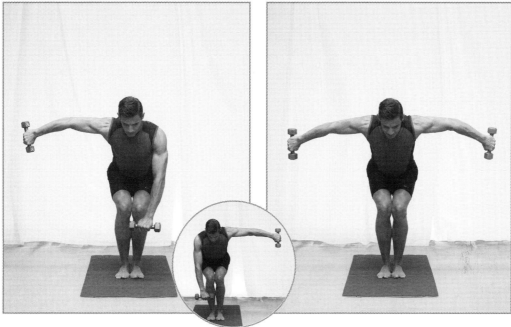

20. Rear Lateral Raise

Engage your right rear delt, inhale, and raise the right dumbbell out to the side to shoulder height. Exhale and press the right dumbbell down to the start position (#19). Make sure to keep your elbow soft and slightly bent through the movement.

21. Repeat #20 with the left dumbbell (see inset).

22. Static Contraction

Inhale and repeat #20 with both dumbbells. Hold the movement at peak contraction. Exhale and then inhale to enhance the peak contraction. Exhale, press both dumbbells down to the start position (#19), and press together the top dumbbell heads.

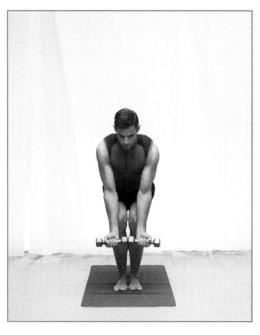

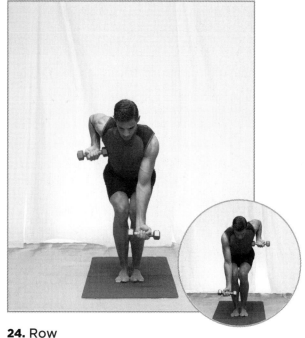

23. Start Position

Rotate your palms to face forward while keeping your elbows slightly bent. Press together the bottom dumbbell heads.

24. Row

Engage your right lat, inhale, and pull the right dumbbell up to your armpit, raising your elbow high above the level of your back. Exhale and press the right dumbbell down to the start position (#23). Think of your hand as a hook, and make sure not to let your right biceps initiate the movement.

25. Repeat #24 with the left dumbbell (see inset).

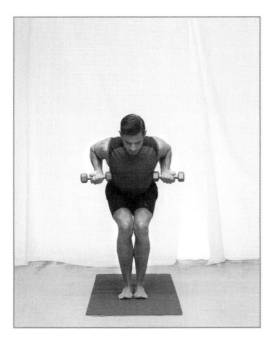

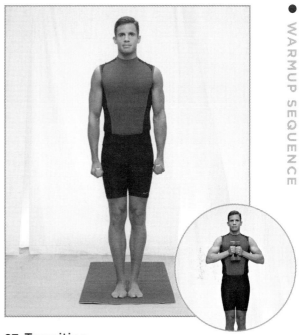

26. Static Contraction

Inhale and repeat #24 with both dumbbells. Hold the movement at peak contraction. Exhale and then inhale to enhance the peak contraction. Exhale, press both dumbbells down to the start position (#23), and press together the bottom dumbbell heads.

27. Transition

Press firmly into your heels and slowly straighten your legs. Gently lift your torso up one vertebra at a time. Round your shoulders up, back, and release down as you return to Mountain pose with dumbbells at your sides.

28. Stand in Mountain pose pressing together both dumbbell heads over your heart (see inset). Hold for 4 breaths.

Chapter 6

IRON YOGA SEQUENCES

After completing the Warmup Sequence, your body should feel ready to begin the main part of the Iron Yoga practice. This chapter includes all of the Iron Yoga sequences—I call it the heart of the practice. As you move through these sequences, remember to apply the principles you learned in Chapter 2. To practice Iron Yoga correctly, you need to make the connections between your mind and muscles—so pay particular attention to the static contractions. Those movements require quite a bit of concentration, but when done correctly over time, you'll really see great body sculpting results. Again, if you don't have time to complete all the sequences in this chapter, make sure you do both right and left sides of any particular sequence.

TREE SEQUENCE—RIGHT LEG

Before balancing on one leg in this sequence, it's helpful to give your legs a rest from the muscle burn you created in Chair pose during the warmup. So this sequence begins in Mountain pose with a Wrist Curl. The wrists and forearms are often neglected in a weight-training program, but development of these body parts is essential—especially for the more challenging upper-body poses performed later in the Sun Salutation. Wrist curls are also excellent for preventing and alleviating carpal tunnel syndrome and other wrist injuries.

Tree pose is the primary yoga pose for this Iron Yoga sequence. In nature, a tree's roots grow deep, and its branches reach to the sky. As you perform Tree pose, keep that image in mind. Your legs and feet represent strong roots; your torso, the trunk; and your arms, the branches. Tree pose is an excellent pose to create symmetry in your body. It requires tremendous mental focus and concentration and is extremely challenging, even without holding dumbbells. Tree pose helps increase lung capacity by expanding your breathing. It also improves steadiness and balance.

At first, you may have trouble balancing. Your mind may wander and lose connection with your body. Plus, the extra weight of the dumbbells adds another challenging dimension to the pose. Don't allow yourself to get frustrated if you have difficulty holding the pose and balancing. Try starting in one of the modified positions; with consistent practice you will improve. As you progress, your nonstanding foot will lift higher up your leg, and strength will increase in the foot, ankle, calf, thigh, and glute of your supported leg. Your body is meant to naturally be in balance. Use your breath and the power of your mind to help you through this sequence.

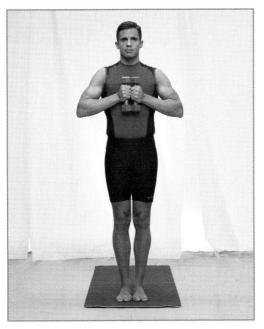

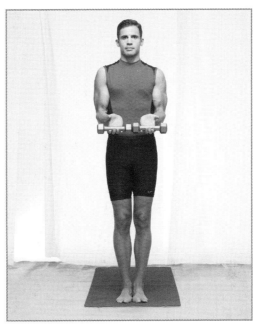

1. Prepare
Stand in Mountain pose, pressing together both dumbbell heads over your heart.

2. Start Position
Place your elbows tightly into the sides of your torso, lower your forearms till they are parallel to the mat with your palms facing upward, and press together the bottom dumbbell heads. Let the dumbbells roll down to your fingertips, so your palms are open and your wrists are curled down.

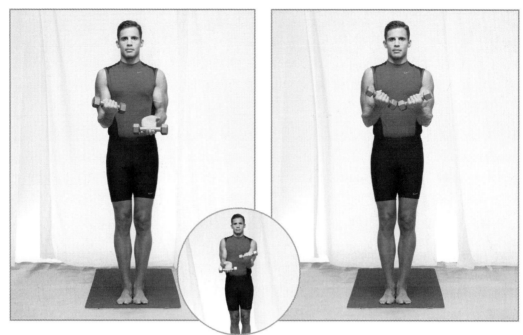

3. Wrist Curl

Engage your right wrist and forearm flexor, inhale, and squeeze the right dumbbell into your right palm. Curl the right dumbbell up and rotate your right wrist back. Exhale and rotate the right dumbbell forward and down to the start position (#2).

4. Repeat #3 with the left dumbbell (see inset).

5. Static Contraction

Inhale and repeat #3 with both dumbbells while pressing together the bottom dumbbell heads. Hold the movement at peak contraction. Exhale and then inhale to enhance the peak contraction. Exhale and rotate both dumbbells forward and down to the start position (#2).

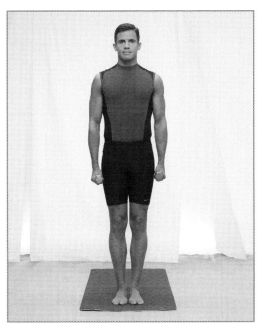

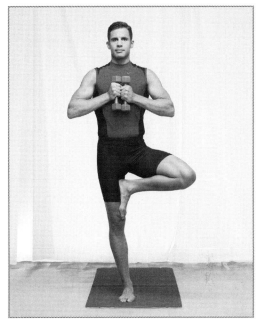

6. Transition

Stand in Mountain pose with the dumbbells at your sides.

7. Tree

Firmly plant your right foot into the mat, pressing into the four corners of the sole of your foot to evenly distribute your weight across the ball of your foot and heel. Think of your heel as the root of a tree. Take a moment to establish this strong foundation because it will greatly assist in your ability to balance. Slowly lift your left knee and press the sole of your left foot against the top of your right inner thigh. If you want, place both dumbbells in your right hand and use your left hand to help lift your left foot into place. Apply equal pressure with your left foot and right inner thigh to create equilibrium in your lower body. Open your left knee out wide. With your right leg active, core engaged, torso tall, and hips and shoulders square, press together both dumbbell heads over your heart. Feel the pressure of both dumbbell heads as strongly as the pressure of your left foot against your right inner thigh. Gaze at a point in front of you that is at eye level. This will help you focus your concentration and steady your balance.

51

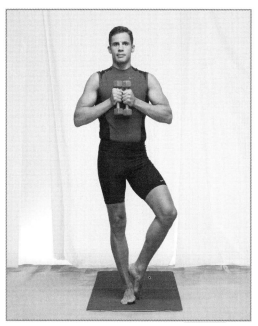

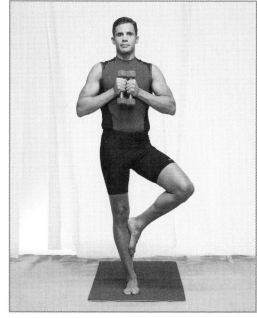

Modifications:

Beginner

Softly place your left toes touching the mat by the inside of your right foot with your left heel pressed into the side of your ankle and shin.

Intermediate

Press your left foot to the inside of your right calf or slightly below your right knee.

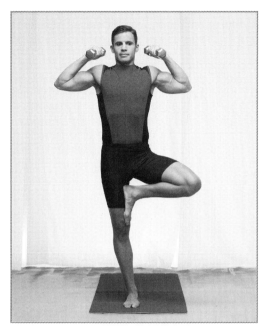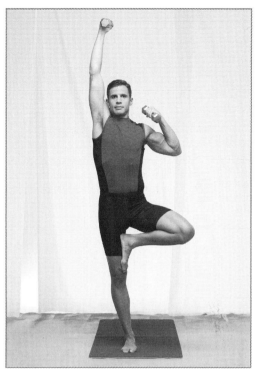

8. Start Position

Bring the dumbbells to your shoulders with your palms facing each other. Extend your elbows out to your sides and back, squeezing your shoulder blades together.

9. Shoulder Overhead Press

Engage your right front and middle delts, inhale, and press the right dumbbell straight overhead. Feel your right biceps pressing close to your right ear at full extension.

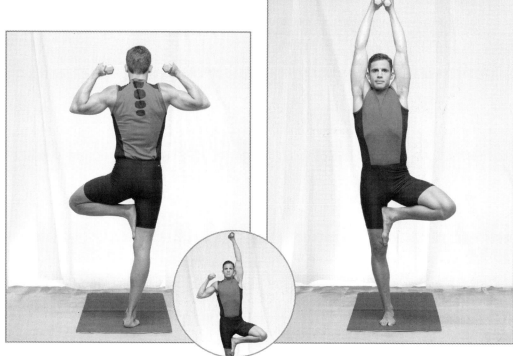

10. Lat Pulldown

Engage your right lat, exhale, and pull down the right dumbbell, keeping your right elbow down, out to your right side, and squeeze back.

11. Repeat #9 and #10 with the left dumbbell (see inset).

12. Static Contraction

Inhale and repeat #9 with both dumbbells. Hold the movement at peak contraction, pressing together both dumbbell heads. Exhale and then inhale to enhance the peak contraction. Exhale and repeat #10 with both dumbbells.

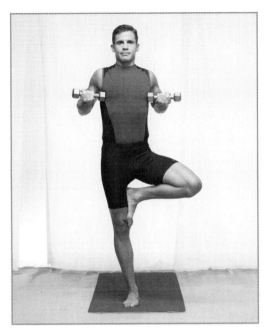

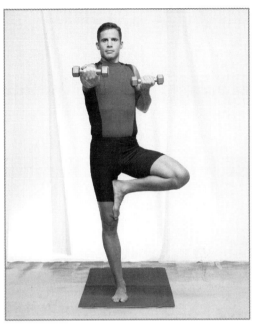

13. Start Position

Place the dumbbells by your armpits with your palms facing upward. Draw your elbows back by squeezing your shoulder blades together.

14. Chest Press

Engage your right pec, inhale, and press the right dumbbell straight forward, keeping your right arm at shoulder height and your right palm facing upward.

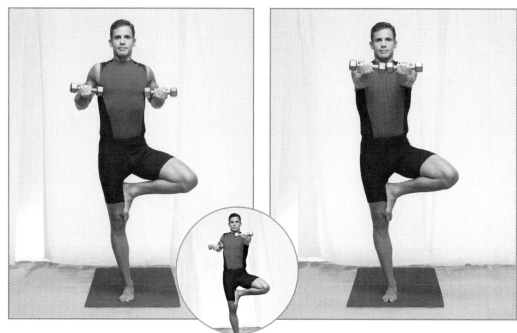

15. Lat Pullback

Engage your right lat, exhale, and pull back the right dumbbell to the side of your chest, keeping your right elbow up and out to your right side, with your right palm facing upward.

16. Repeat #14 and #15 with the left dumbbell (see inset).

17. Static Contraction

Inhale and repeat #14 with both dumbbells and press together the bottom dumbbell heads at full extension. Hold the movement at peak contraction. Exhale and then inhale to enhance the peak contraction. Exhale and repeat #15 with both dumbbells.

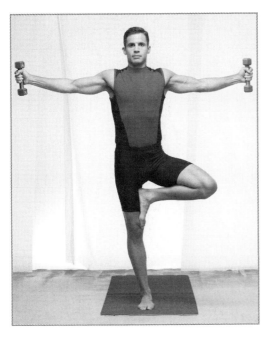

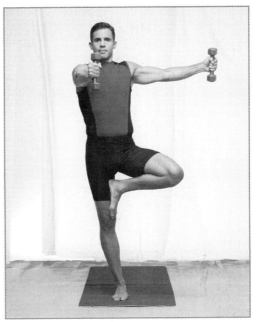

18. Start Position

Extend both dumbbells straight out to your sides at shoulder height and rotate your palms to face forward.

19. Chest Flye

Engage your right pec, inhale, and press the right dumbbell forward and across to the front centerline of your body. Keep your right arm straight and at shoulder height through the full range of motion.

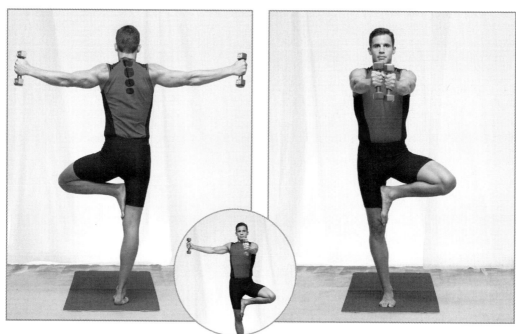

20. Reverse Flye

Engage your right rear delt and lat, exhale, and pull the right dumbbell out to your right side and back.

21. Repeat #19 and #20 with the left dumbbell (see inset).

22. Static Contraction

Inhale and repeat #19 with both dumbbells. Hold the movement at peak contraction, pressing together both dumbbell heads. Exhale and then inhale to enhance the peak contraction. Exhale and repeat #20 with both dumbbells.

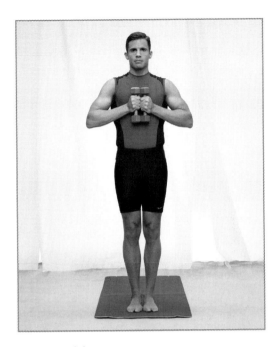

23. Transition

Stand in Mountain pose, pressing together both dumbbell heads over your heart. Hold for 4 breaths.

TREE SEQUENCE—LEFT LEG

Before working your left leg in Tree pose, it's beneficial to rest in Mountain pose. This helps you refocus and take a mental break after the challenge of balancing on one leg and performing the compound weight-training exercises for the upper body. It's also a great time to work the other sides of your wrists and forearms by doing the Reverse Wrist Curl. The External/Internal Rotation is the first time you'll be targeting your rotator cuff muscle group. This movement helps to keep your shoulders healthy by improving strength, flexibility, and range of motion.

After working both legs in Tree pose, your lower body will feel incredibly symmetrical and balanced. Don't be surprised if you find one leg stronger than the other. It is very common to have a more dominant side that is more easily able to balance and hold the pose. If you've had a prior foot, ankle, or knee injury, this will also make balancing more difficult. To correct this imbalance, focus greater attention on the weaker side. Creating equilibrium in the body is one of the best ways to protect yourself from injury.

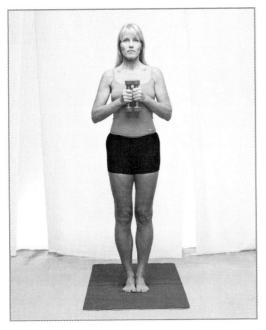

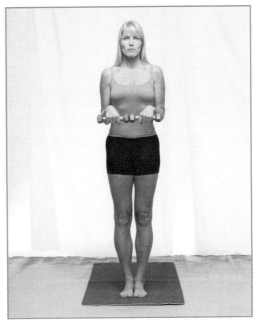

1. Prepare

Stand in Mountain pose, pressing together both dumbbell heads over your heart.

2. Start Position

Place your elbows tightly into the sides of your torso, lower your forearms till they are parallel to the mat with your palms facing downward, and press together the top dumbbell heads. Curl your wrists to a downward position and let the dumbbells roll down to your fingertips.

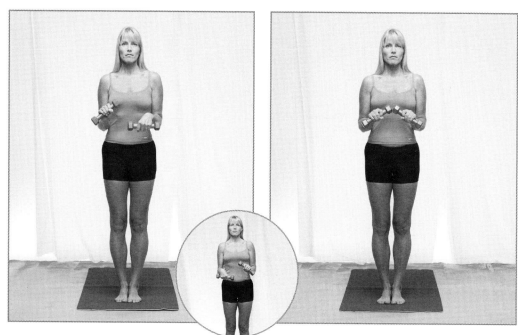

3. Reverse Wrist Curl

Engage your right wrist and forearm extensor, inhale, and squeeze the right dumbbell into your right palm. Curl the right dumbbell up and rotate your right wrist back. Exhale and rotate the right dumbbell forward and down to the start position (#2).

4. Repeat #3 with the left dumbbell (see inset).

5. Static Contraction

Inhale and repeat #3 with both dumbbells while pressing together the top dumbbell heads. Hold the movement at peak contraction. Exhale and then inhale to enhance the peak contraction. Exhale and rotate both dumbbells forward and down to the start position (#2).

6. Transition

Stand in Mountain pose with the dumbbells at your sides.

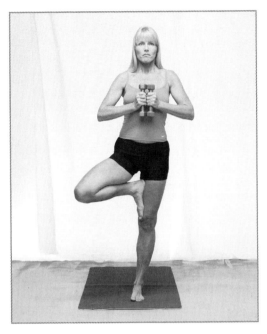

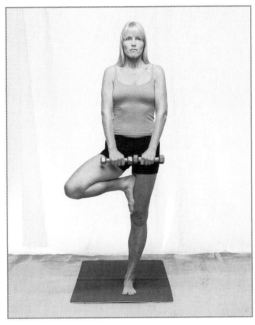

7. Tree

Firmly plant your left foot into the mat, pressing into the four corners of the sole of your foot to evenly distribute your weight across the ball of your foot and heel. Think of your heel as the root of a tree. Take a moment to establish this strong foundation because it will greatly assist in your ability to balance. Slowly lift your right knee and press the sole of your right foot against the top of your left inner thigh. If you want, place both dumbbells in your left hand and use your right hand to help lift your right foot into place. Apply equal pressure with your right foot and left inner thigh to create equilibrium in your lower body. Open your right knee out wide. With your left leg active, core engaged, torso tall, and hips and shoulders square, press together both dumbbell heads over your heart. Feel the pressure of both dumbbell heads as strongly as the pressure of your right foot against your left inner thigh. Gaze at a point in front of you that is at eye level. This will help you focus your concentration and steady your balance. (See Tree pose modifications on page 52.)

8. Start Position

Lower the dumbbells down in front of your thighs with your palms facing your body and the top dumbbell heads pressing together.

63

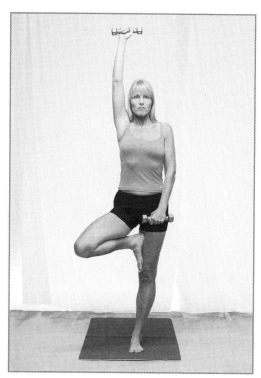

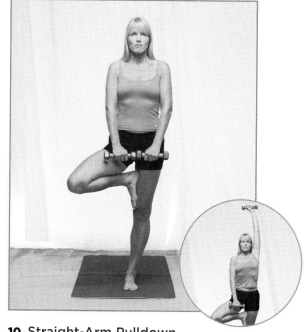

9. Front Raise

Engage your right front delt, inhale, and raise the right dumbbell straight up the front centerline of your body, over the crown of your head. Press your right biceps close to your right ear at full extension. Keep your right wrist and elbow soft to make sure your right front delt does all the work.

10. Straight-Arm Pulldown

Engage your right lat and pec, exhale, and pull down the right dumbbell over the front of your head (think pulling over a barrel) and down to your thigh. Keep your arm straight through the full range of motion.

11. Repeat #9 and #10 with the left dumbbell (see inset).

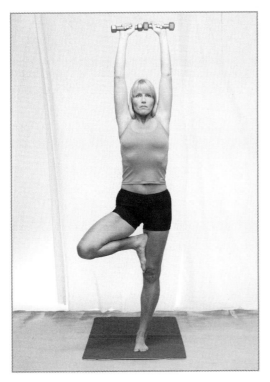

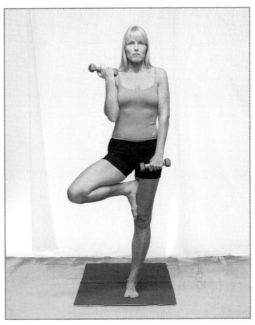

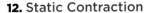

12. Static Contraction

Inhale and repeat #9 with both dumbbells while pressing together the top dumbbell heads. Hold the movement at peak contraction. Exhale and then inhale to enhance the peak contraction. Exhale and repeat #10 with both dumbbells while pressing together the top dumbbell heads.

13. Biceps Curl

Engage your right biceps, inhale, and rotate your right palm to face upward, then curl the right dumbbell up to your shoulder. At the top of the movement, rotate your right wrist outward, so the bottom dumbbell head points to your right shoulder. This twist will help to sculpt your biceps.

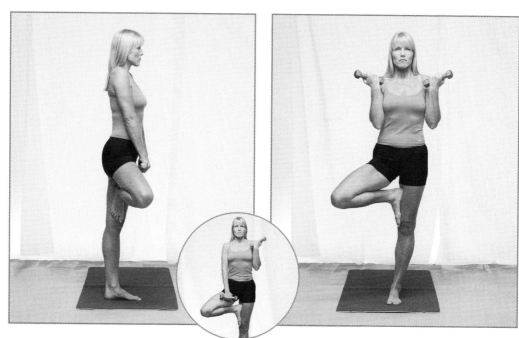

14. Triceps Pressdown

Engage your right triceps, exhale, and rotate your right palm to face downward, then press the right dumbbell down to your thigh.

15. Repeat #13 and #14 with the left dumbbell (see inset).

16. Static Contraction

Inhale and repeat #13 with both dumbbells. Hold the movement at peak contraction. Exhale and then inhale to enhance the peak contraction. Exhale and repeat #14 with both dumbbells while pressing together the top dumbbell heads.

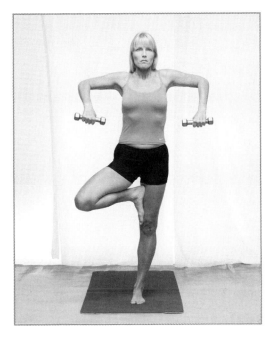

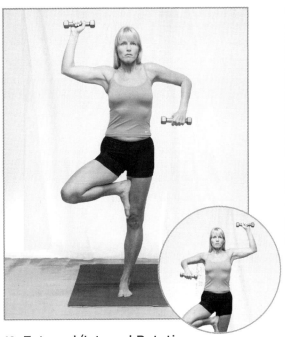

17. Start Position

Raise your arms so your elbows are at shoulder height. Position the dumbbells under your elbows, with your forearms perpendicular to the mat and your palms facing backward.

18. External/Internal Rotation

Engage your right rotator cuff, inhale, and raise the right dumbbell forward and up, rotating over your right shoulder and squeezing back at the top of the movement. Exhale and lower the right dumbbell forward and down, rotating under your right shoulder and squeezing back at the bottom of the movement.

19. Repeat #18 with the left dumbbell (see inset).

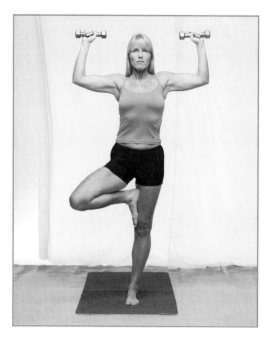

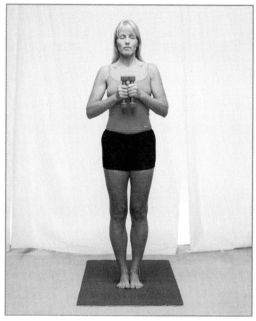

20. Static Contraction

Inhale and repeat #18 with both dumbbells. Hold the movement at peak contraction. Exhale and then inhale to enhance the peak contraction. Exhale and lower both dumbbells to the start position (#17).

21. Stand in Mountain pose, pressing together both dumbbell heads over your heart, and softly close your eyes.

POWER LUNGE SEQUENCE—RIGHT LEG

The Power Lunge Sequence includes four yoga poses. The sequence starts off in Triangle pose, a classic standing yoga pose, which aligns and energizes your spine. It also strengthens your legs, hips, ankles, and feet. From Triangle, you'll flow into Warrior 2, named after a legendary Hindu warrior. This pose helps to alleviate stiffness in your neck and shoulders while expanding your chest and lungs. Side Angle Lunge and Crescent Lunge continue to strengthen your legs.

This series will provide an intense muscle burn in your legs and create tremendous leg muscular endurance. Make sure to use your breath to take you deep into each pose, but never sacrifice form and proper alignment and never create joint pain. Use your feet to press in opposite directions as if separating the yoga mat. When you start to feel a burn in your legs, use your exhalation to breathe through the burn and relax your body. Visualize your legs becoming toned and sculpted.

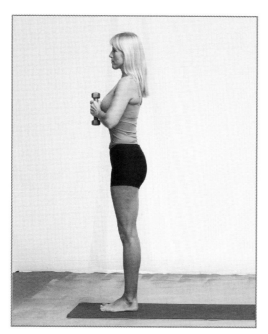

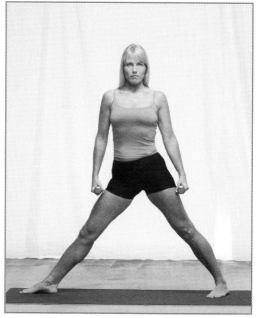

1. Prepare

Stand in Mountain pose, pressing together both dumbbell heads over your heart.

2. Transition

Lower the dumbbells to your sides. Step back with your left leg about 3 to 4 feet. Turn your left foot in about 15° and keep your right foot pointed forward. Make sure to maintain a straight line from heel to heel. Rotate your torso to the left to square your hips and shoulders over the center of your body.

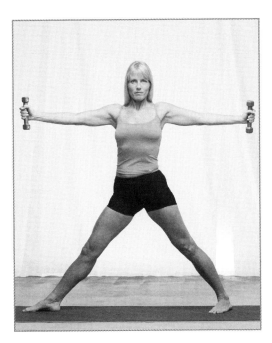

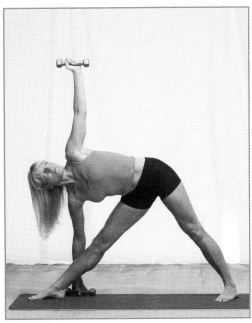

3. Transition

Inhale and raise your arms straight out to your sides to shoulder height. Exhale and rotate the dumbbells so that your palms are facing the left side. Your wrists should be directly over your ankles. Activate your legs, keeping them straight, and engage your core.

4. Triangle

Inhale to prepare, exhale, and lean your torso and the right dumbbell forward over your right leg. Contract your right oblique and lower the right dumbbell down to the mat outside your right heel. Raise the left dumbbell above your left shoulder, creating one straight line of energy from dumbbell to dumbbell. Turn your head up and gaze over the left dumbbell, opening your left shoulder and the left side of your chest. On each exhalation, challenge your upper body by reaching your arms in opposite directions. Separate the mat by pressing your feet in opposite directions, using the four corners of your right foot and outer side of your left foot. This will greatly tone your calves, inner thighs, and glutes. Hold for 4 breaths.

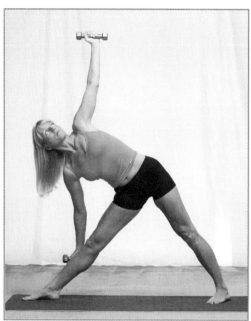
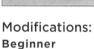
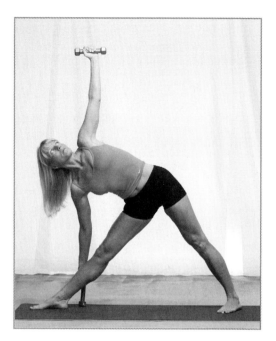

Modifications:

Beginner

Lower the right dumbbell to the outside of your right calf. On each exhalation, try to lower the right dumbbell closer to the mat.

Intermediate

Use the right dumbbell as a block for support by standing it on the mat outside your right heel. Softly touch the top of the right dumbbell with your right fingertips. On each exhalation, try to lower your right fingertips closer to the mat.

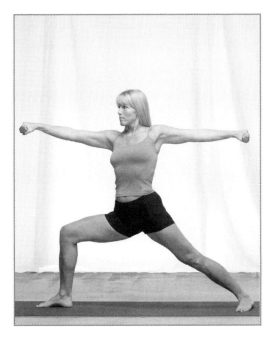 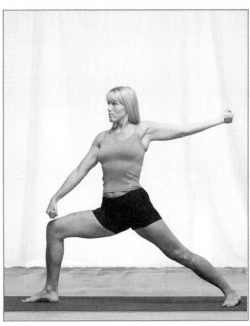

5. Warrior 2

From Triangle pose, inhale and contract your left oblique to lift your torso center over your hips. Bring your arms straight out to your sides to shoulder height, palms facing downward. Bend your right knee 90° over your ankle in line with your second and third toes. Your right thigh should be parallel to the mat, and your left leg should remain straight and active. Keep your torso centered, with your hips and shoulders square. Turn your head to the right and gaze over the right dumbbell.

6. Start Position

Lower the right dumbbell to your right knee with your right palm facing down to prepare for a Lateral Raise. Keep your left arm straight at shoulder height and rotate your left palm to face upward to prepare for a Biceps Curl. Keep your torso tall and don't lean forward over your right leg. If you have any knee injuries, don't bend your right knee as far as shown above.

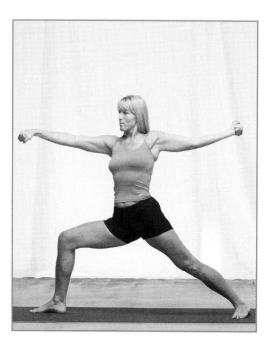 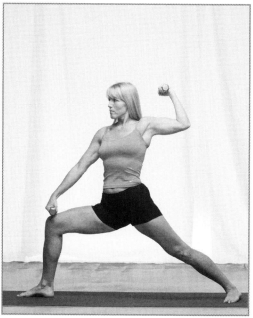

7. Lateral Raise

Engage your right middle delt, inhale, and raise the right dumbbell to shoulder height, keeping your wrist and elbow soft. Exhale and press the right dumbbell down to the start position (#6).

8. Biceps Curl

Engage your left biceps, inhale, and curl the left dumbbell toward your shoulder. Exhale and press the left dumbbell back to the start position (#6).

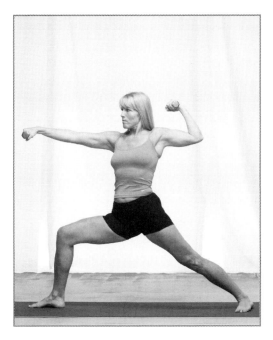

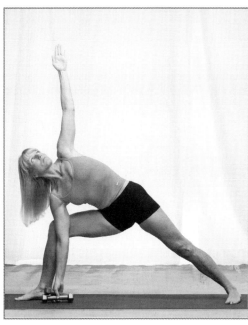

9. Static Contraction

Inhale and repeat #7 and #8 with both dumbbells. Hold the movement at peak contraction. Exhale and then inhale to enhance the peak contraction. Exhale and return both dumbbells to the start position (#6).

10. Transition

From Warrior 2 pose, lower the right dumbbell to your right heel. Plant your right elbow on the inside of your right knee. Place both dumbbells together in your right hand. Rotate your left shoulder up and raise your left arm straight up over your left shoulder, opening the left side of your chest. Turn your head and gaze over your left fingertips.

Modification:

Use only one dumbbell in your right hand and place the other one on the mat next to you.

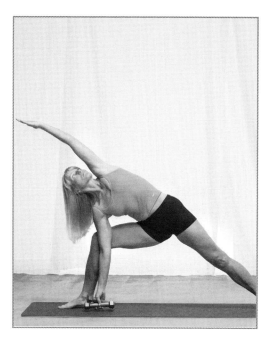

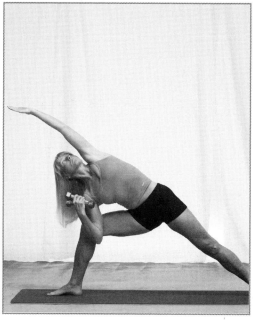

11. Side Angle Lunge/Start Position

Inhale to prepare, and as you exhale, extend your left arm straight forward over the left side of your head with your left biceps pressing toward your left ear. Keep your right knee bent over your right ankle and press into the four corners of your right foot. Keep your left leg straight and active. Try to maintain a straight line from your left heel to your left fingertips. Maintain your gaze over your left biceps.

12. Concentration Curl

Engage your right biceps, inhale, and curl the right dumbbells to your right shoulder. Exhale and press the right dumbbells down to the start position (#11).

13. Repeat #12.

14. Static Contraction

Inhale and repeat #12. Hold the movement at peak contraction. Exhale and then inhale to enhance the peak contraction. Exhale and press the right dumbbells down to the start position (#11).

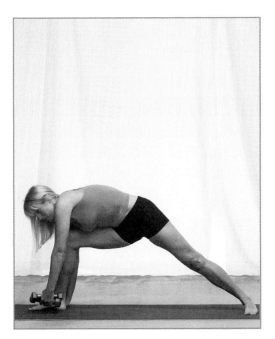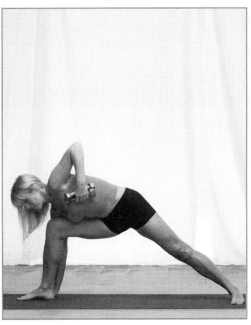

15. Start Position

Bring your left arm forward, place both dumb-bells in your left hand reaching low to the mat in front of you. Place your right fingertips or palm softly on the mat outside your right foot.

16. Single-Arm Row

Engage your left lat, inhale, and pull the left dumbbells up to your armpit, raising your elbow high above the level of your back. Exhale and press the left dumbbells down to the start position (#15).

17. Repeat #16.

18. Static Contraction

Inhale and repeat #16. Hold the movement at peak contraction. Exhale and then inhale to enhance the peak contraction. Exhale and press the left dumbbells down to the start position (#15).

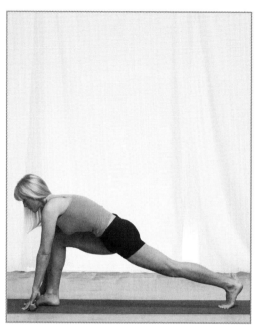

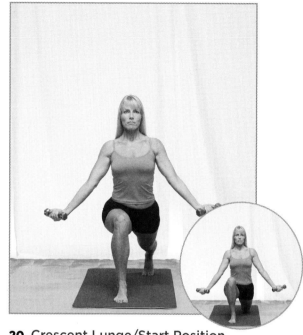

19. Power Lunge

From Side Angle Lunge pose, lower the dumbbells to the mat on each side of your right foot and place your fingertips softly on the mat, with your hands shoulder-width apart. Lift your left heel off the mat and rotate your left foot so your toes are curled and facing forward. Step back 2 to 3 inches with your right foot, so that it is between your hands and your right knee is bent over your ankle. Square your torso and hips to face forward. Release your shoulders down and back away from your ears to alleviate any tension from your neck and upper back and feel your spine long. Press into the four corners of your right foot to activate your calf, hamstring, and glute of your right leg. Keep your left leg straight and active as you press down and back into your left heel, feeling a great stretch in your hip flexor, quad, and groin of your left leg. Hold for 4 breaths.

20. Crescent Lunge/Start Position

From the Power Lunge pose, take hold of a dumbbell in each hand and bring them to your right thigh. Raise your torso up center and gently arch your lower back. Keep your right knee bent 90° over your right ankle with your right thigh parallel to the mat. Lift your chest and keep your shoulders square. Bring the dumbbells down to your sides with your palms facing outward.

Modification:

Lower your left knee to the mat and press the top of your left foot into the mat or bring your left foot slightly forward (see inset).

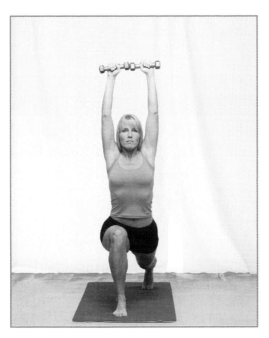 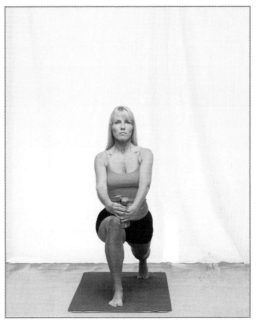

21. Full Overhead Lateral Raise

Engage your middle delts, inhale, and raise the dumbbells straight out to your sides, with your palms facing upward. Extend your arms overhead, pressing together the top dumbbell heads. Exhale and press the dumbbells down to your sides, palms facing downward, to the start position (#20).

22. Repeat #21.

23. Static Contraction

Inhale and repeat #21. Hold the movement at peak contraction, pressing together the top dumbbell heads. Exhale and then inhale to enhance the peak contraction. Exhale and press the dumbbells down to your sides, palms facing downward, to the start position (#20).

24. Start Position

Bring your arms straight in front of your waist and hold the dumbbells together in your hands.

79

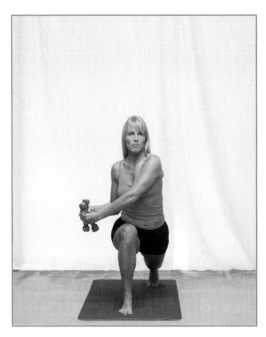

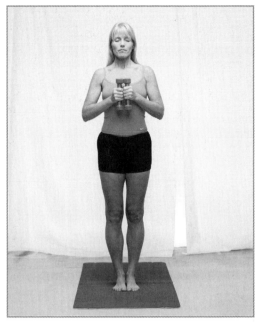

25. Oblique Twist

Engage your right oblique, inhale, and rotate your torso to the right side. Bend your right elbow back while keeping your left arm straight. Keep your head in a neutral position and gaze forward. Exhale and rotate your torso forward to the start position (#24).

26. Repeat #25.

27. Static Contraction

Inhale and repeat #25. Hold the movement at peak contraction. Exhale and then inhale to enhance the peak contraction. Exhale and rotate your torso forward to the start position (#24).

28. Stand in Mountain pose, pressing together both dumbbell heads over your heart, and softly close your eyes. Hold for 4 breaths.

SUN SALUTATION SEQUENCE I

The Sun Salutation Sequence is one of the most well-known series of poses in yoga. Just about every style of yoga tradition incorporates some version of the Sun Salutation. As with all of the sequences in Iron Yoga, each movement in the Sun Salutation is synchronized to the breath. Usually, the Sun Salutation Sequence is performed at the beginning of your yoga practice. I've included the sequence here to give your body and mind a rest from the Power Lunge Sequence on your right side and before we begin a similar sequence on your left side. As you perform the Sun Salutation, pay close attention to the rhythm of your breathing. In Plank, Chaturanga, Upward-Facing Dog, and Downward-Facing Dog, hold the pose for 4 breaths. Enjoy the flowing movement of this series as it brings you increased flexibility and strength for the entire body. This series of movements is particularly important to improve circulation and develop respiratory and cardiovascular health.

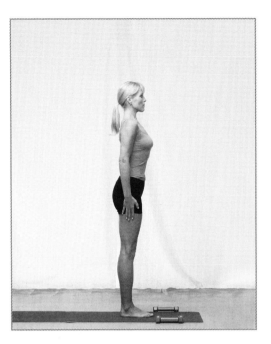

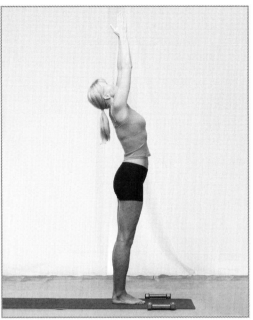

1. Prepare

Stand in Mountain pose, bend your knees, and gently lower the dumbbells to the mat by your sides. Resume Mountain pose with your arms by your sides.

2. Mountain Back Bend

Inhale and raise your arms straight out to your sides and high overhead. Lift your chest and lean your torso backward, pressing together your palms. Gaze over your fingertips.

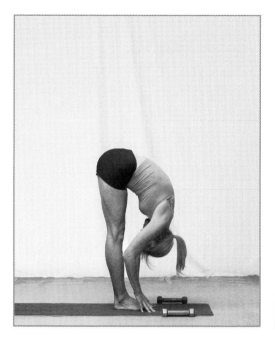

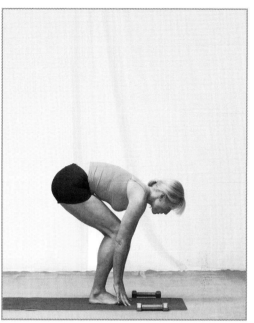

3. Standing Forward Bend

Exhale and dive forward and down. Fold your torso over your thighs, tuck your chin to your chest, lower your forehead toward your knees or shins, and reach your fingertips to the mat by the sides of your toes.

4. Transition

Inhale to prepare for Plank pose by softly bending your knees and lifting your head up.

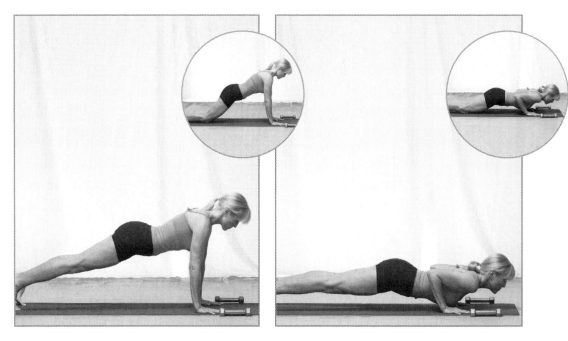

5. Plank (High Pushup)

Exhale and either jump both legs back or step back one leg at a time. Curl your toes into the mat, pressing your heels back with your feet hip-width apart. Align your hands under your shoulders, with your fingers spread wide, and release your shoulders down and back away from your ears. Create one straight line of energy from the crown of your head to your heels, with your arms and legs straight, hips even, back flat, head neutral, and gaze slightly forward. Activate your lower back, glutes, and legs. Engage your core. This is an excellent pose to develop strength in your shoulders, arms, chest, and abdominal region. Hold for 4 breaths.

Modification:

Anytime the pose becomes too intense, lower softly to your knees, keeping your arms straight (see inset). If you can, raise your knees off the mat every other breath. Gradually, with consistency, your upper-body strength will increase.

6. Chaturanga (Low Pushup)

From Plank pose, inhale to prepare, and as you exhale, bend your elbows to lower your body 2 to 3 inches from the mat. Press your elbows into the sides of your torso and keep your shoulders down and back away from your ears. Shift your head and upper body slightly forward, so your elbows are at the midpoint of your torso and your upper arms are parallel to the mat. Keep your legs straight and active with your heels pressing back. Engage your core. Maintain a flat back and long spine with a straight line of energy from the crown of your head to your heels. Lift your head slightly up and gaze forward. This pose requires tremendous strength and works every muscle group in your body. Hold for 4 breaths.

Modification:

If this pose is too difficult, lower softly to your knees (see inset). Keep your elbows bent and your torso 2 to 3 inches off the mat. If you can, raise your knees off the mat every other breath.

84

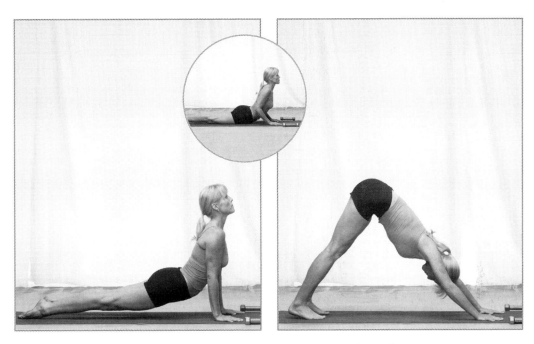

7. Upward-Facing Dog

From Chaturanga pose, inhale and press the tops of your feet into the mat and straighten your arms, keeping your wrists under your shoulders while you lift up your chest and head. Open your shoulders wide and arch your lower back. Release your shoulders down and back away from your ears. Engage your lower back and core while activating your glutes and legs. Hold for 4 breaths.

Modification:

Keep your legs on the mat and softly bend your elbows (see inset). Use the strength of your lower back to keep your torso off the mat. (This modification is also called Cobra pose.)

8. Downward-Facing Dog

From Upward-Facing Dog, exhale and lift your tailbone high to create an inverted "V" with your body. Press your armpits toward your knees, your chest toward your thighs, and your heels down to the mat. Keep your head neutral and your back flat, with your spine long. Keep your arms and legs straight and active. Make sure your feet are hip-width apart, with your toes spread wide. Check your hands to make sure they are shoulder-width apart, with your fingers spread wide. Rotate your inner elbows toward each other to open your shoulders and improve your flexibility and range of motion. Press into the knuckles of your index fingers to relieve any strain that may develop in your hands, wrists, and forearms. Feel a straight line of energy from your tailbone to your fingertips and your tailbone to your heels. Downward-Facing Dog is one of the few yoga poses that increases the strength of the entire body, while at the same time stretching and relaxing the entire body. Hold for 4 breaths.

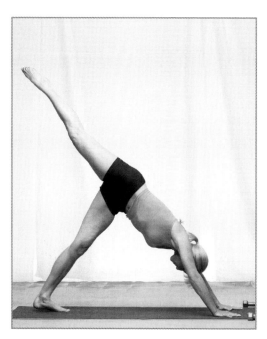

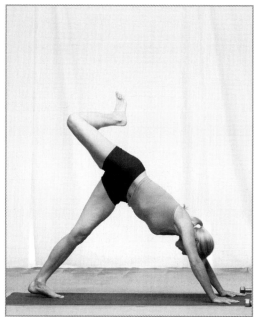

9. Split-Leg Downward-Facing Dog

Inhale and raise your right foot off the mat, extending your right leg high. Keep your right leg straight and active. Try to create a straight line of energy from your right fingertips to your right toes. Point your right toes to create length, then exhale and flex your right foot.

10. Leg Curl

Engage your right hamstring and glute, inhale, and curl your right heel to your butt. Exhale and press your right heel back to full extension. Lower your right foot back to the mat.

11. Repeat #9 and #10 with your left leg.

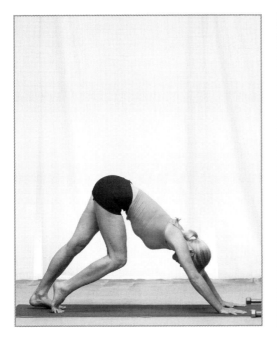

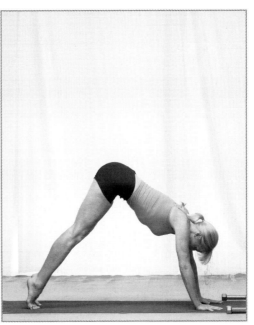

12. Transition

Inhale and bend your right knee softly to give your right leg a rest. Exhale and press your left heel down to the mat to get a good stretch for the back of your left leg. Repeat on the other side.

13. Transition

Press both of your heels down, inhale, and lift high up on your toes. Feel your tailbone lift higher and lean your torso forward, with your head over your hands. Exhale and press your heels back down to the mat, getting a deeper stretch for the back of your legs.

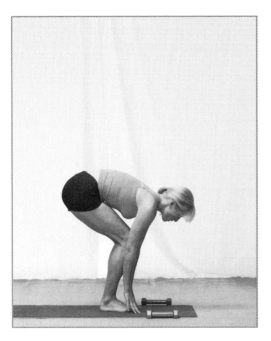

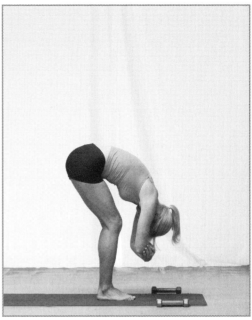

14. Transition

Inhale to prepare, exhale, and either jump both legs forward or step forward one leg at a time to your hands.

15. Rag Doll

Keep your knees softly bent, fold your torso over your thighs, tuck your chin to your chest and lower your forehead to your knees or shins. Place your fingertips on your opposite elbows. Use your breath to create total relaxation throughout your body. Gently shake your head "no" from right to left a couple of times, alleviating any tension, tightness, and stress from your neck, shoulders, and upper back. Gently nod your head "yes" a couple of times. Hold for 4 breaths. On an exhalation, release your fingertips from your elbows and lower them to the mat in front of your toes.

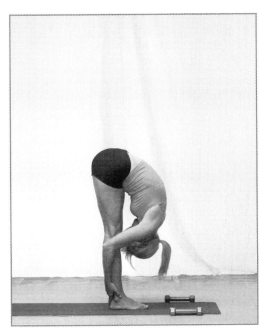

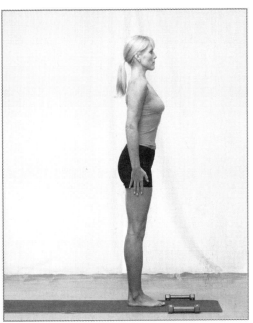

16. Standing Forward Bend

Walk your fingertips behind your heels and gently hold the backs of your ankles. Inhale to prepare, exhale, and press firmly into your heels, lifting your knees to straighten and activate your legs. Lift your tailbone higher and feel a tremendous stretch throughout the Achilles tendons, calves, hamstrings, and lower back. Use your exhale breath to extend your torso lower and stretch deeper. This pose is excellent to relieve any lower back pain and discomfort and terrific for opening the hamstrings to improve flexibility and range of motion.

17. Mountain

Inhale to prepare, exhale, release your hands from the backs of your ankles, and place your fingertips in front of your toes. Very slowly walk your fingertips up the fronts of your legs, lifting your torso one vertebra at a time. Keep your legs active and, as your torso lifts to waist level, engage your core. Round your shoulders up, back, and release them down, returning to Mountain pose, with your arms at your sides.

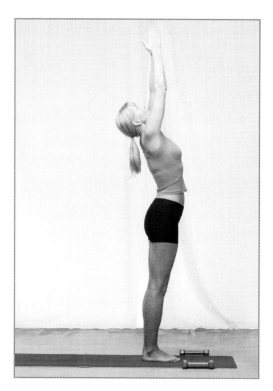

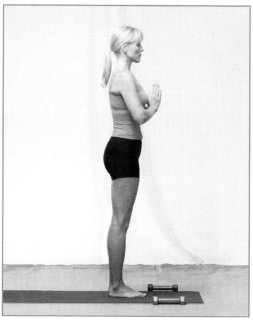

18. Mountain Back Bend

Inhale and raise your arms straight out to your sides and high overhead. Lift your chest and lean your torso backward, pressing together your palms. Gaze over your fingertips.

19. Mountain Hands over Heart

Exhale, lower your arms down to your sides, and gently press your palms together over your heart. Softly close your eyes and connect with your breath. Take a moment to feel the strength and positive energy you created throughout your full body. Feel your breath deeper, your body stronger, and your mind more relaxed. Hold for 4 breaths.

POWER LUNGE SEQUENCE—LEFT LEG

Here you will be repeating the Power Lunge Sequence on your left side. Again, you may feel that one side is stronger than the other. That's fine. As you continue your Iron Yoga practice, you will develop symmetry between your right and left sides. The one modification you will be making in this sequence on your left side is that you'll perform a Chest Pullover instead of a Full Overhead Lateral Raise while in Crescent Lunge pose.

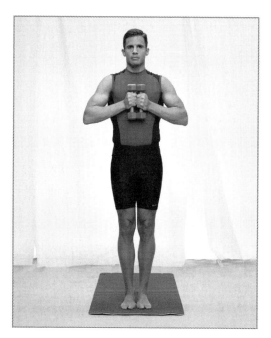

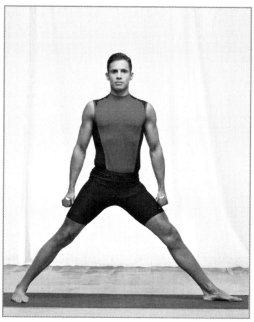

1. Prepare

Stand in Mountain pose, pressing together both dumbbell heads over your heart.

2. Transition

Lower the dumbbells to your sides. Step back with your right leg about 3 to 4 feet. Turn your right foot in about 15° and keep your left foot pointed forward. Make sure to maintain a straight line from heel to heel. Rotate your torso to the right to square your hips and shoulders over the center of your body.

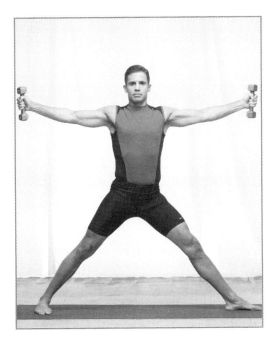

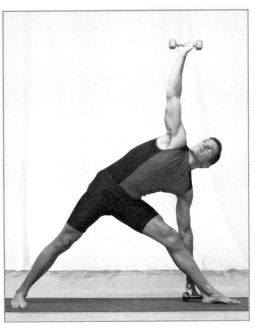

3. Transition

Inhale and raise your arms straight out to your sides to shoulder height. Exhale and rotate the dumbbells, so that your palms are facing the right side. Your wrists should be directly over your ankles. Activate your legs, keeping them straight, and engage your core.

4. Triangle

Inhale to prepare, exhale, and lean your torso and the left dumbbell forward over your left leg. Contract your left oblique and lower the left dumbbell down to the mat outside your left heel. Raise the right dumbbell above your right shoulder, creating one straight line of energy from dumbbell to dumbbell. Turn your head up and gaze over the right dumbbell, opening your right shoulder and the right side of your chest. On each exhalation, challenge your upper body by reaching your arms in opposite directions. Separate the mat by pressing your feet in opposite directions, using the four corners of your left foot and outer side of your right foot. This will greatly tone your calves, inner thighs, and glutes. Hold for 4 breaths.

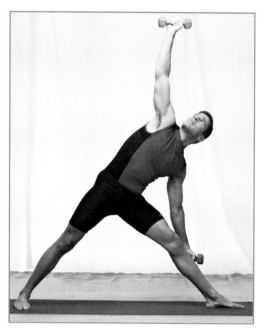 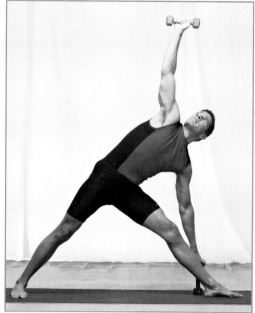

Modifications:

Beginner

Lower the left dumbbell to the outside of your left calf. On each exhalation, try to lower the left dumbbell closer to the mat.

Intermediate

Use the left dumbbell as a block for support by standing it on the mat outside your left heel. Softly touch the top of the left dumbbell with your left fingertips. On each exhalation, try to lower your left fingertips closer to the mat.

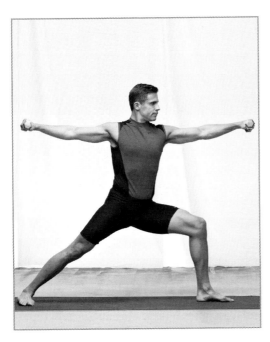

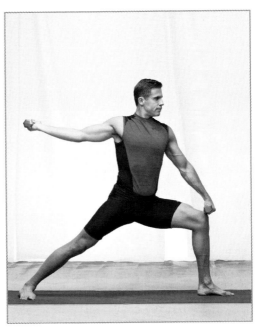

5. Warrior 2

From Triangle pose, inhale and contract your right oblique to lift your torso over your hips. Bring your arms straight out to your sides to shoulder height, palms facing downward. Bend your left knee 90° over your ankle in line with your second and third toes. Your left thigh should be parallel to the mat, and your right leg should remain straight and active. Keep your torso centered, with your hips and shoulders square. Turn your head to the left and gaze over the left dumbbell.

6. Start Position

Lower the left dumbbell to your left knee, with your left palm facing down to prepare for a Lateral Raise. Keep your right arm straight at shoulder height and rotate your right palm to face upward to prepare for a Biceps Curl. Keep your torso tall and don't lean forward over your left leg. If you have any knee injuries, don't bend your left knee as far as shown above.

95

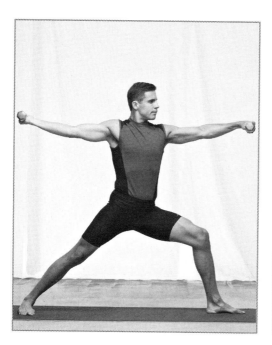

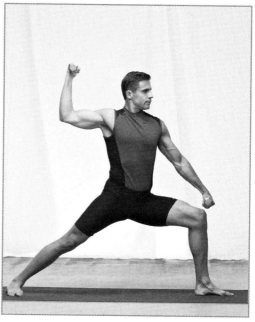

7. Lateral Raise

Engage your left middle delt, inhale, and raise the left dumbbell to shoulder height, keeping your wrist and elbow soft. Exhale and press the left dumbbell down to the start position (#6).

8. Biceps Curl

Engage your right biceps, inhale, and curl the right dumbbell toward your shoulder. Exhale and press the right dumbbell back to the start position (#6).

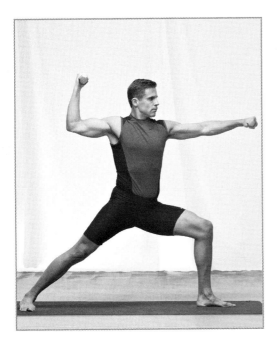 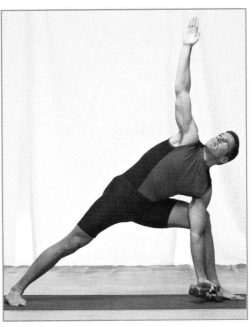

9. Static Contraction

Inhale and repeat #7 and #8 with both dumb-bells. Hold the movement at peak contraction. Exhale and then inhale to enhance the peak contraction. Exhale and return both dumbbells to the start position (#6).

10. Transition

From Warrior 2 pose, lower the left dumbbell to your left heel. Plant your left elbow on the inside of your left knee. Place both dumbbells together in your left hand. Rotate your right shoulder up and raise your right arm straight up over your right shoulder, opening the right side of your chest. Turn your head and gaze over your right fingertips.

Modification:

Hold only one dumbbell in your left hand and place the other one on the mat next to you.

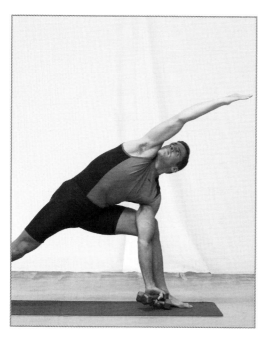

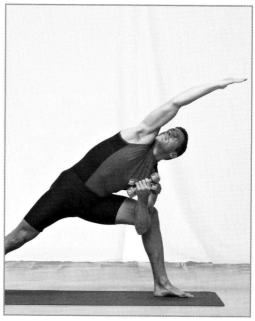

11. Side Angle Lunge/Start Position

Inhale to prepare, and as you exhale, extend your right arm straight forward over the right side of your head, with your right biceps pressing toward your right ear. Keep your left knee bent over your left ankle and press into the four corners of your left foot. Keep your right leg straight and active. Try to maintain a straight line from your right heel to your right fingertips. Maintain your gaze over your right biceps.

12. Concentration Curl

Engage your left biceps, inhale, and curl the left dumbbells to your left shoulder. Exhale and press the left dumbbells down to the start position (#11).

13. Repeat #12.

14. Static Contraction

Inhale and repeat #12. Hold the movement at peak contraction. Exhale and then inhale to enhance the peak contraction. Exhale and press the left dumbbells down to the start position (#11).

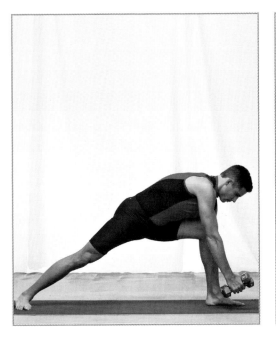
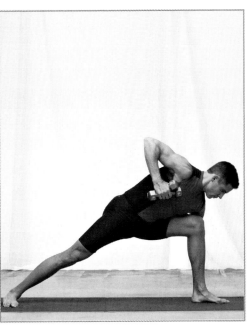

15. Start Position

Bring your right arm forward and place both dumbbells in your right hand, reaching low to the mat in front of you. Place your left fingertips or palm softly on the mat outside your left foot.

16. Single-Arm Row

Engage your right lat, inhale, and pull the right dumbbells up to your armpit, raising your elbow high above the level of your back. Exhale and press the right dumbbells down to the start position (#15).

17. Repeat #16.

18. Static Contraction

Inhale and repeat #16. Hold the movement at peak contraction. Exhale and then inhale to enhance the peak contraction. Exhale and press the right dumbbells to the start position (#15).

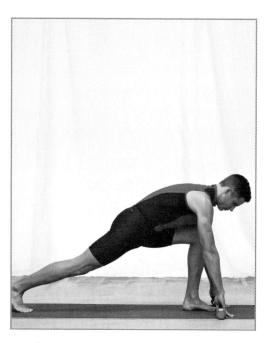

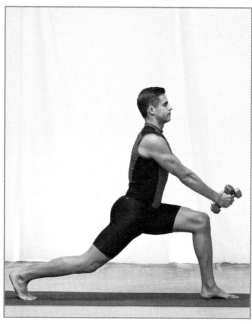

19. Power Lunge

From Side Angle Lunge pose, lower the dumbbells to the mat on each side of your left foot and place your fingertips softly on the mat, with your hands shoulder-width apart. Lift your right heel off the mat and rotate your right foot so that your toes are curled and facing forward. Step back 2 to 3 inches with your left foot, so that it is between your hands and your left knee is bent over your ankle. Square your torso and hips to face forward. Release your shoulders down and back away from your ears to alleviate any tension from your neck and upper back and feel your spine long. Press into the four corners of your left foot to activate your calf, hamstring, and glute of your left leg. Keep your right leg straight and active as you press down and back into your right heel, feeling a great stretch in your hip flexor, quad, and groin of your right leg. Hold for 4 breaths.

20. Crescent Lunge/Start Position

From Power Lunge pose, take hold of a dumbbell in each hand and bring them to your left thigh. Raise your torso up center and gently arch your lower back. Keep your left knee bent 90° over your left ankle with your left thigh parallel to the mat. Lift your chest and keep your shoulders square. Bring your arms straight in front of your waist, with your hands holding the dumbbells together.

Modification:

Lower your right knee to the mat and press the top of your right foot into the mat, or bring your right foot slightly forward. (See photo inset on page 78.)

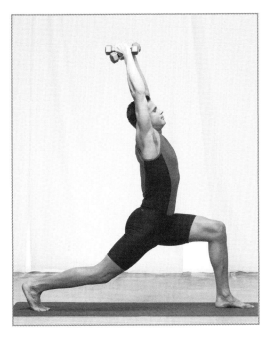

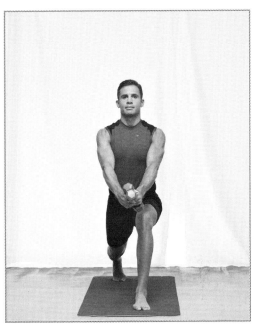

21. Chest Pullover

Engage your pecs and front delts, inhale, and raise the dumbbells up the front centerline of your body over the crown of your head and pull back. Exhale and pull the dumbbells over the crown of your head and down the front centerline of your body, returning to the start position (#20). Keep your arms straight through the full range of motion.

22. Repeat #21.

23. Static Contraction

Inhale and repeat #21. Hold the movement at peak contraction. Exhale and then inhale to enhance the peak contraction. Exhale and pull the dumbbells over the crown of your head and down to the start position (#20).

24. Start Position

Maintain your arms straight in front of your waist, with your hands holding the dumbbells together.

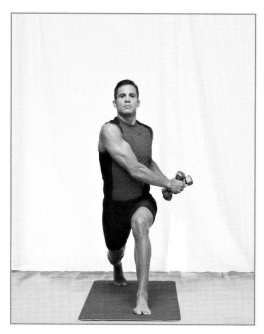

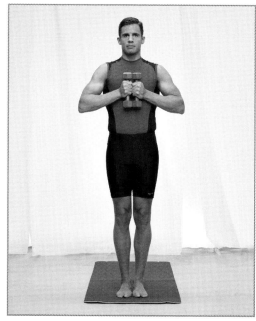

25. Oblique Twist

Engage your left oblique, inhale, and rotate your torso to the left side. Bend your left elbow back while keeping your right arm straight. Keep your head in a neutral position and gaze forward. Exhale and rotate your torso forward to the start position (#24).

26. Repeat #25.

27. Static Contraction

Inhale and repeat #25. Hold the movement at peak contraction. Exhale and then inhale to enhance the peak contraction. Exhale and rotate your torso forward to the start position (#24).

28. Stand in Mountain pose, pressing together both dumbbell heads over your heart. Hold for 4 breaths.

SINGLE-LEG BALANCE SEQUENCE—RIGHT LEG

This is one of the most challenging sequences in the Iron Yoga workout. The sequence starts off with Half Moon and Standing Back Bend poses to give your body and mind a rest from the Power Lunge Sequence you just completed on your left leg. Half Moon tones your obliques and stretches your torso, arms, and shoulders. If you like to swim, it will improve your "streamlined" position in the water. Standing Back Bend pose will invigorate your lower back.

The next three poses in this sequence will further improve your balance, concentration, and mental focus. Warrior 3 pose helps to tone your abs and strengthen and sculpt your legs. Standing Leg Raise pose creates an equal balance of strength in your quads and hamstrings, which is so important in keeping your knee joints healthy.

Eagle pose takes its name from the stature and grace of this beautiful and majestic bird. The intertwining position of the legs helps to strengthen your calves and ankles. You may want to first try the weight-training movements in Eagle without the dumbbells a few times. Then, as you increase your strength, add the weights.

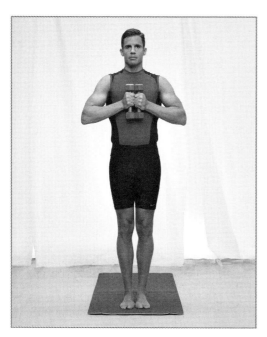

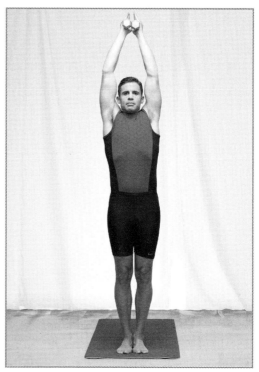

1. Prepare

Stand in Mountain pose, pressing together both dumbbell heads over your heart.

2. Start Position

Inhale and press the dumbbells straight over-head while pressing together both dumbbell heads. Feel your biceps close to your ears at full extension. Exhale and rotate your palms, so your knuckles are facing upward. Inhale and reach your fingertips higher. Make sure to keep your legs active and your core engaged.

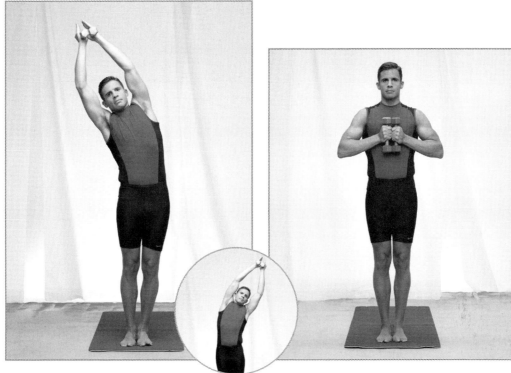

3. Half Moon

Engage your right oblique, inhale to prepare, exhale, and lean your torso to the right side. Press your heels firmly into the mat, keeping your legs and arms straight. You should feel a great stretch along the left side of your body. Hold for 4 breaths. On each exhalation, contract your right oblique stronger and extend your torso farther to the right.

4. Repeat #3, leaning to your left side (see inset).

5. Transition

Stand in Mountain pose, pressing together both dumbbell heads over your heart.

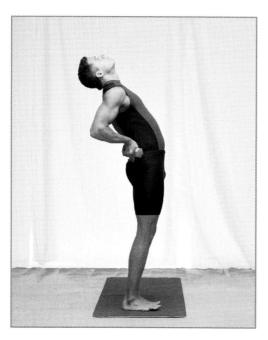

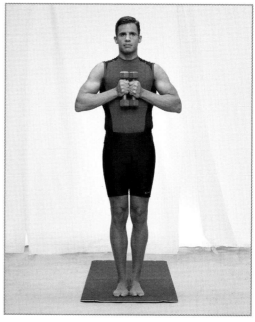

6. Standing Back Bend

Gently place your palms and dumbbells into your lower back. Squeeze your shoulder blades together and bring your elbows back. Inhale to prepare, exhale, and gently start leaning your torso and your head backward. Open your shoulders and chest wide. As you press firmly into your heels, lift your toes to get a stretch for your shins and the soles of your feet. On each exhalation, try to extend and lean back farther. This should feel great in your lower back area. Hold for 4 breaths.

7. Transition

Stand in Mountain pose, pressing together both dumbbell heads over your heart.

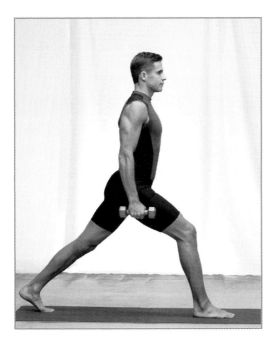 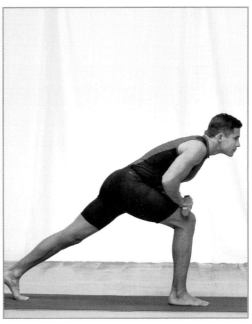

8. Transition

Lower the dumbbells to your sides. Plant your right foot firmly into the mat. Feel the four corners of your right foot to set up a strong foundation. Step back 3 to 4 feet with your left foot. Stand softly on your left toes, with your left heel off the mat and your left leg straight and active.

9. Transition

Bend your right knee over your ankle and fold your torso over your right thigh. Keep your back flat and your spine long.

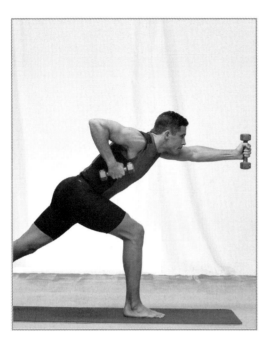

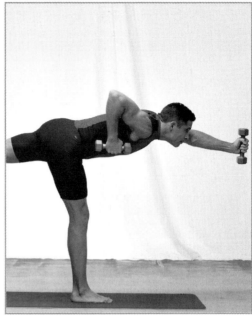

10. Transition

Bring the right dumbbell to your right armpit, with your right elbow lifted up. Raise the left dumbbell straight forward to shoulder height, with your palm facing right. Lift your head slightly and gaze at a point in front of you or keep your head neutral and gaze at a point on the mat. This will assist you in maintaining your balance.

11. Warrior 3

Inhale to prepare, exhale, and lift your left foot off the mat and extend your left leg straight back, pointing your toes. Try to create one straight line of energy from the left dumbbell to your left toes. Straighten your right leg and keep your torso parallel to the mat.

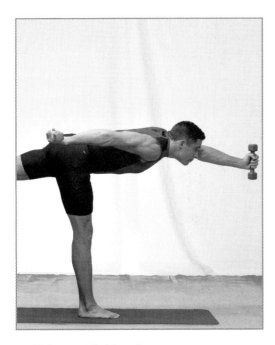

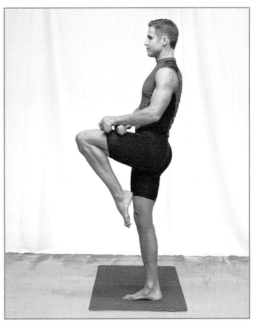

12. Triceps Kickback

Engage your right triceps, inhale, and press back the right dumbbell. At full extension, rotate your right palm to face upward. This twist will help to sculpt your triceps.

13. Biceps Curl

Engage your right biceps, exhale, and curl the right dumbbell to your armpit.

14. Repeat #12 and #13.

15. Static Contraction

Inhale and repeat #12. Hold the movement at peak contraction. Exhale and then inhale to enhance the peak contraction. Exhale and repeat #13.

16. Standing Leg Raise

From Warrior 3 pose, lower the left dumbbell down to your side and raise your torso to an upright and tall position. Lift your left knee to waist level with your left thigh parallel to the mat and your left toes pointing downward. Release your shoulders down and back away from your ears, engage your core, and keep your right leg straight and active. Place both dumbbells on top of your left thigh to add resistance.

Modification:

For additional support, you can try this pose standing next to a wall or holding on to a chair with your right hand.

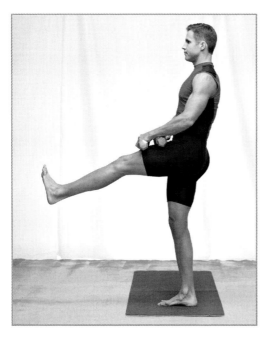

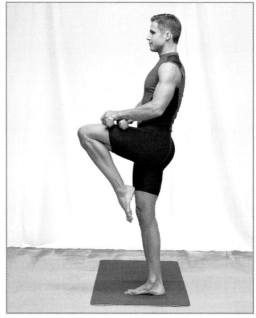

17. Leg Extension

Engage your left quad, inhale, and extend your left lower leg straight forward and flex your left foot, so your toes are pointing upward.

18. Leg Curl

Engage your left hamstring, exhale, and curl your left lower leg back, pointing your toes to the mat.

19. Repeat #17 and #18.

20. Static Contraction

Inhale and repeat #17. Hold the movement at peak contraction. Exhale and then inhale to enhance the peak contraction. Exhale and repeat #18.

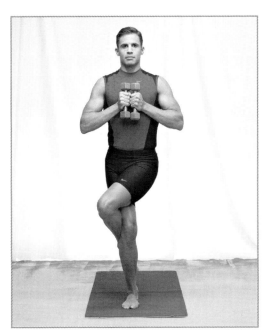

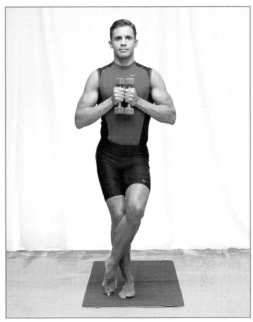

21. Eagle

From Standing Leg Raise pose, bend your right knee and slide your left heel down the outside of your right knee, crossing your left leg over your right leg. Extend your left foot out to the right side and back. Try to hook your left foot behind your right calf and lock your left toes around your right ankle. Sit low and deep into your glutes to challenge your right leg. Keep your torso tall, hips square, core engaged, and shoulders released down and back away from your ears. Press together both dumbbell heads over your heart. Gaze at a point in front of you that is at eye level to assist you with balance.

Modifications:
Beginner

Eagle pose is a very challenging single-leg balancing pose. If you're just starting your Iron Yoga practice and have trouble balancing or getting into the pose, try crossing your left leg over your right leg and placing your left toes softly on the mat to assist you.

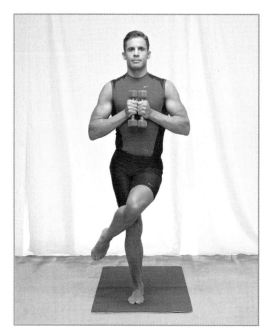

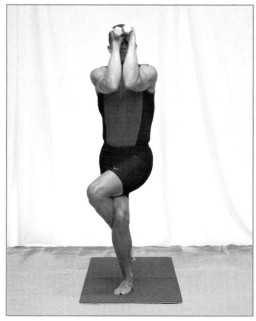

Intermediate

Raise your left foot off the mat, but don't hook it behind your right calf. For both modifications, make sure to sit low and deep into your glutes to get the full sculpting benefit for your right leg.

22. Start Position

Lift the top dumbbell heads up in front of your forehead with your palms facing each other. Press together both dumbbell heads and squeeze together your elbows.

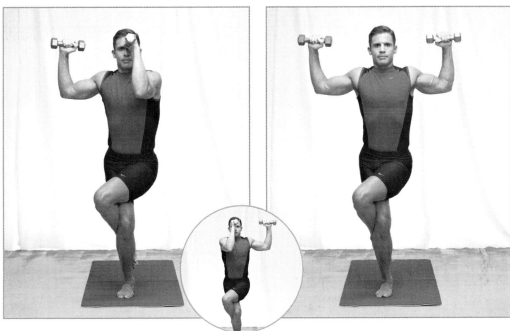

23. Reverse Flye

Engage your right rear delt and lat, inhale, and pull the right dumbbell out to your right side and back, keeping your elbow bent and your forearm perpendicular to the mat through the full range of motion.

24. Chest Flye

Engage your right pec, exhale, and press the right dumbbell forward and across to the front centerline of your body. Press together both dumbbell heads and squeeze together your elbows.

25. Repeat #23 and #24 with the left dumbbell (see inset).

26. Static Contraction

Inhale and repeat #23 with both dumbbells. Hold the movement at peak contraction. Exhale and then inhale to enhance the peak contraction. Exhale and repeat #24 with both dumbbells.

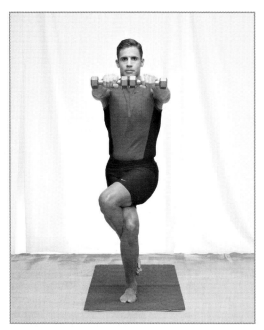

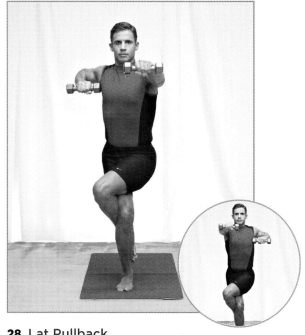

27. Start Position

Extend both dumbbells straight forward to shoulder height and rotate your palms to face downward. Press together the top dumbbell heads.

28. Lat Pullback

Engage your right lat, inhale, and pull back the right dumbbell to the side of your chest, keeping your right elbow up and out to your right side with your right palm facing downward.

29. Chest Press

Engage your right pec, exhale, and press the right dumbbell straight forward, keeping your right arm at shoulder height and your right palm facing downward.

30. Repeat #28 and #29 with the left dumbbell. (See inset.)

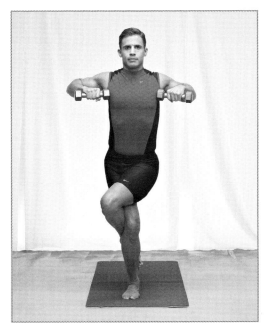 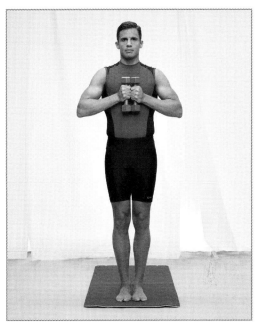

31. Static Contraction

Inhale and repeat #28 with both dumbbells. Hold the movement at peak contraction. Exhale and then inhale to enhance the peak contraction. Exhale and repeat #29 with both dumbbells. Press together the top dumbbell heads at full extension.

32. Stand in Mountain pose, pressing together both dumbbells over your heart. Hold for 4 breaths.

SINGLE-LEG BALANCE SEQUENCE—LEFT LEG

In this sequence, you will be repeating Warrior 3, Standing Leg Raise, and Eagle poses with the left leg. The sequence starts off in Mountain pose with a Calf Raise to give your body and mind a rest from the challenging Single-Leg Balance Sequence you just completed on your right leg. Calf Raise is an excellent exercise to help you develop strength in your calves, ankles, feet, and toes. Strength in the lower leg is very important for performing all of the single-leg balancing poses in Iron Yoga. A second variation of the External/Internal Rotation here will strengthen your rotator cuffs and increase flexibility and range of motion for your shoulders. The Knee Lift and Dancer's poses at the end will give your lower body a good stretch after the challenges of this sequence.

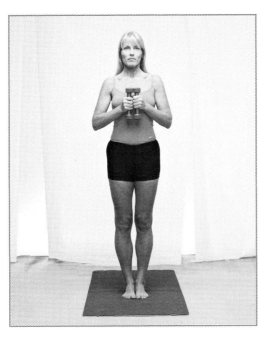

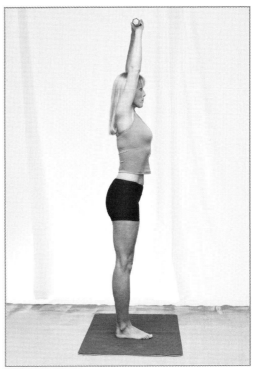

1. Prepare

Stand in Mountain pose, pressing together both dumbbell heads over your heart.

2. Start Position

Inhale and press the dumbbells straight overhead while pressing together both dumbbell heads. Feel your biceps close to your ears at full extension. Exhale, and rotate your palms to face forward and press together the top dumbbell heads. Make sure to keep your legs active and your core engaged.

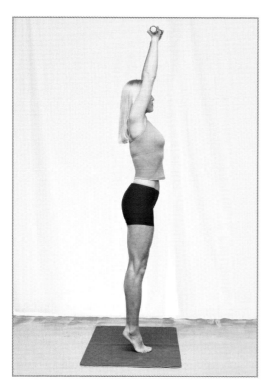

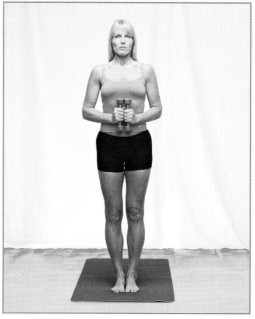

3. Calf Raise

Engage your calves, inhale to prepare, exhale, and lift your heels 1 inch off the mat, coming up onto your toes and the balls of your feet. On each exhalation, challenge yourself to lift your heels 1 inch higher and squeeze your calves tighter. Hold for 4 breaths.

4. Start Position

Stand in Mountain pose, pressing together both dumbbell heads over your navel.

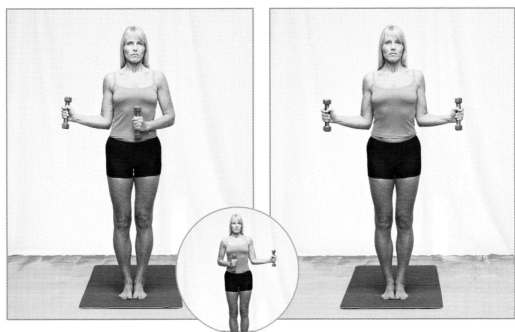

5. External/Internal Rotation

Engage your right rotator cuff, inhale, and pull the right dumbbell out to your right side, rotating your shoulder and squeezing the right dumbbell back. Exhale and press the right dumbbell forward, rotating your shoulder and pressing together both dumbbell heads over your navel.

6. Repeat #5 with the left dumbbell (see inset).

7. Static Contraction

Inhale and repeat #5 with both dumbbells. Hold the movement at peak contraction. Exhale and then inhale to enhance the peak contraction. Exhale and press both dumbbells forward to the start position (#4).

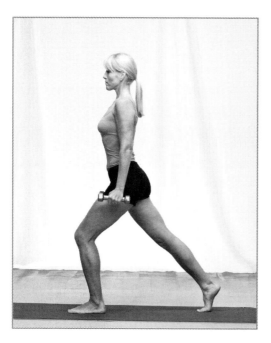

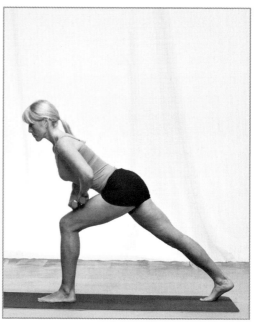

8. Transition

Lower the dumbbells to your sides. Plant your left foot firmly into the mat. Feel the four corners of your left foot to set up a strong foundation. Step back 3 to 4 feet with your right foot. Stand softly on your right toes, with your right heel off the mat and your right leg straight and active.

9. Transition

Bend your left knee over your ankle and fold your torso over your left thigh. Keep your back flat and your spine long.

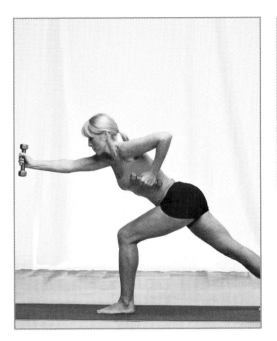 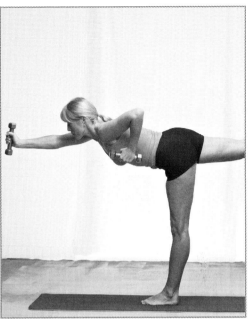

10. Transition

Bring the left dumbbell to your left armpit with your left elbow lifted up. Raise the right dumbbell straight forward to shoulder height with your palm facing left. Lift your head slightly and gaze at a point in front of you or keep your head neutral and gaze at a point on the mat. This will assist you in maintaining your balance.

11. Warrior 3

Inhale to prepare, exhale, and lift your right foot off the mat and extend your right leg straight back, pointing your toes. Try to create one straight line of energy from the right dumbbell to your right toes. Straighten your left leg and keep your torso parallel to the mat.

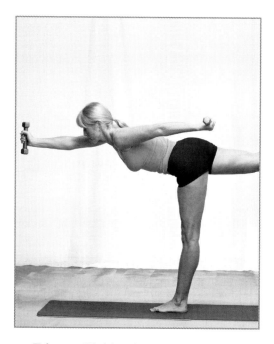

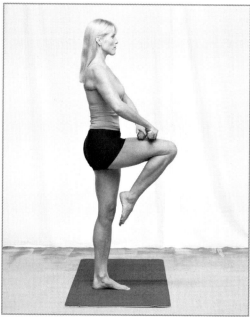

12. Triceps Kickback

Engage your left triceps, inhale, and press back the left dumbbell. At full extension, rotate your left palm to face upward. This twist will help to sculpt your triceps.

13. Biceps Curl

Engage your left biceps, exhale, and curl the left dumbbell to your armpit.

14. Repeat #12 and #13.

15. Static Contraction

Inhale and repeat #12. Hold the movement at peak contraction. Exhale and then inhale to enhance the peak contraction. Exhale and repeat #13.

16. Standing Leg Raise

From Warrior 3 pose, lower the right dumbbell down to your side and raise your torso to an upright and tall position. Lift your right knee to waist level with your right thigh parallel to the mat and your right toes pointing downward. Release your shoulders down and back away from your ears, engage your core, and keep your left leg straight and active. Place both dumbbells on top of your right thigh to add resistance.

Modification:

For additional support, you can try this pose standing next to a wall or holding on to a chair with your left hand.

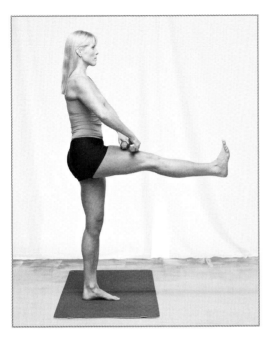

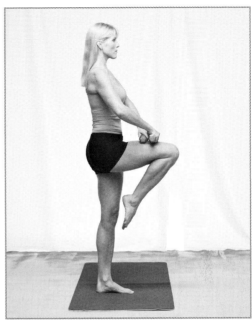

17. Leg Extension

Engage your right quad, inhale, and extend your right lower leg straight forward and flex your right foot, so your toes are pointing upward.

18. Leg Curl

Engage your right hamstring, exhale, and curl your right lower leg back, pointing your toes to the mat.

19. Repeat #17 and #18.

20. Static Contraction

Inhale and repeat #17. Hold the movement at peak contraction. Exhale and then inhale to enhance the peak contraction. Exhale and re-peat #18.

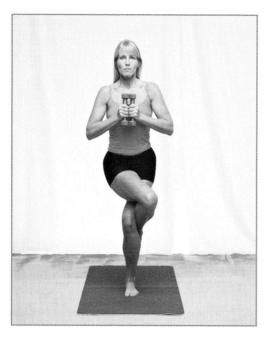

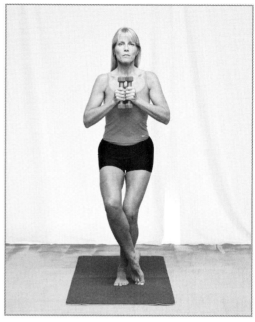

21. Eagle

From Standing Leg Raise pose, bend your left knee and slide your right heel down the outside of your left knee, crossing your right leg over your left leg. Extend your right foot out to the left side and back. Try to hook your right foot behind your left calf and lock your right toes around your left ankle. Sit low and deep into your glutes to challenge your left leg. Keep your torso tall, hips square, core engaged, and shoulders released down and back away from your ears. Press together both dumbbell heads over your heart. Gaze at a point in front of you that is at eye level to assist you with balance.

Modifications:
Beginner

Eagle pose is a very challenging single-leg balancing pose. If you're just starting your Iron Yoga practice and have trouble balancing or getting into the pose, try crossing your right leg over your left leg and placing your right toes softly on the mat to assist you.

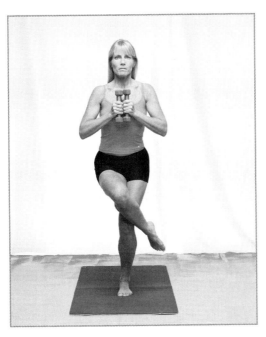

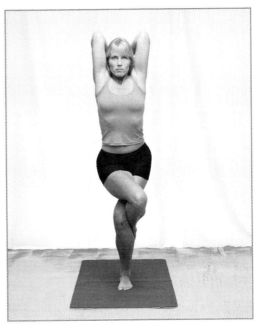

Intermediate

Raise your right foot off the mat, but don't hook the right foot behind your left calf. For both modifications, make sure to sit low and deep into your glutes to get the full sculpting benefit for your left leg.

22. Start Position

Raise both dumbbells overhead while pressing together both dumbbell heads and lower the top dumbbell heads down to the back portion of your neck. Point your elbows up and press your biceps to your ears.

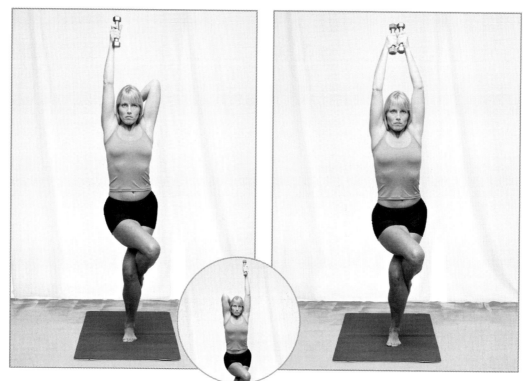

23. Triceps Overhead Extension

Engage your right triceps, inhale, and raise the right dumbbell straight overhead. Press your right biceps close to your right ear at full extension. Exhale and curl the right dumbbell down to the start position (#22).

24. Repeat #23 with the left dumbbell (see inset).

25. Static Contraction

Inhale and repeat #23 while pressing together both dumbbell heads. Hold the movement at peak contraction. Exhale and then inhale to enhance the peak contraction. Exhale and curl both dumbbells down to the start position (#22).

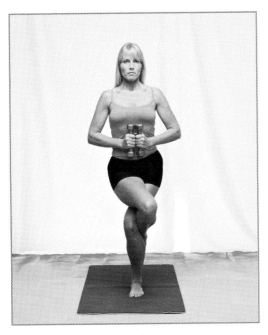

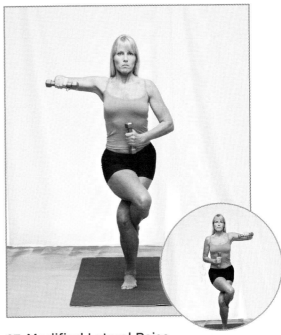

26. Start Position

Separate the dumbbells and lower your elbows to each side. Press together both dumbbell heads over your navel.

27. Modified Lateral Raise

Engage your right middle delt, inhale, and raise the right dumbbell out to your right side, keeping your right elbow bent and lifting to shoulder height. Engage your right pec, exhale, and press the right dumbbell down to the start position (#26), pressing together both dumbbell heads.

28. Repeat #27 with the left dumbbell (see inset).

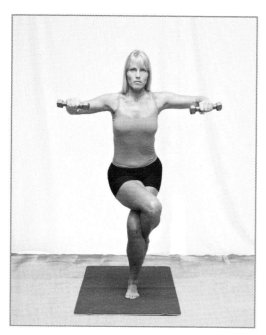

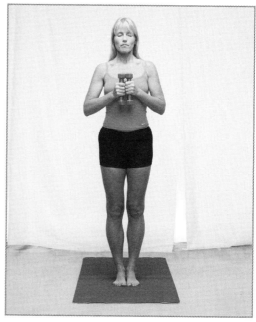

29. Static Contraction

Inhale and repeat #27 with both dumbbells. Hold the movement at peak contraction. Exhale and then inhale to enhance the peak contraction. Exhale and press both dumbbells down to the start position (#26), pressing together both dumbbell heads over your navel.

30. Transition

Stand in Mountain pose, pressing together both dumbbell heads over your heart and softly close your eyes. Hold for 4 breaths.

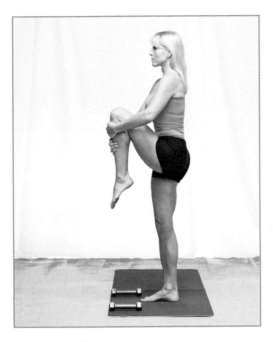

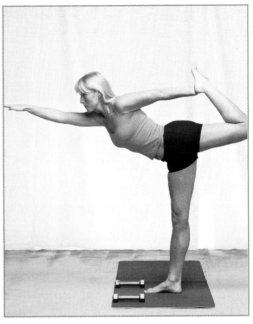

31. Knee Lift

Bend your knees and gently lower the dumbbells to the mat by your sides. Firmly plant your right foot into the mat. Inhale and lift your left knee to your chest. Point your left toes to the mat and squeeze your shoulder blades together. Hold for 4 breaths.

32. Dancer's Pose

Release your left knee, taking hold of your left inner ankle with your left hand, and extend your right arm forward at shoulder height. Inhale to prepare, and on your exhalation, lean your torso forward and gently lift your left foot and heel back and up. Gaze over your right fingertips. This is a great stretch for your left quad and hip flexor. Hold for 4 breaths.

33. Repeat #31 and #32 with your right leg.

SUN SALUTATION SEQUENCE 2

This is the second Sun Salutation Sequence. You repeat this sequence here to further stretch your body and prepare for the floor poses in the next chapter. In this Sun Salutation Sequence, you will hold each movement for only 1 breath, so there should be a more steady flow from one pose to the next. In the first Sun Salutation, you held each of the poses for 4 breaths to increase strength in your upper body. Remember to let your breath control the flow of the movement. At the end of the sequence, you should feel exhilarated and refreshed.

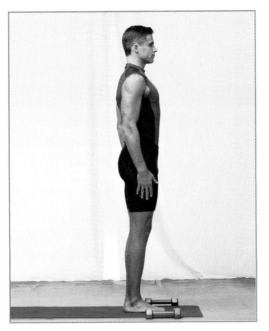

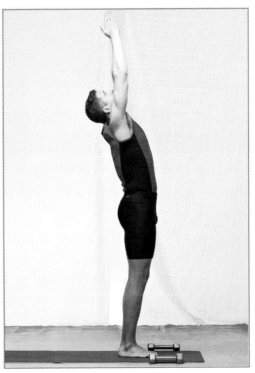

1. Prepare

Stand in Mountain pose, with your arms by your sides.

2. Mountain Back Bend

Inhale and raise your arms straight out to your sides and high overhead. Lift your chest and lean your torso backward, pressing together your palms. Gaze over your fingertips.

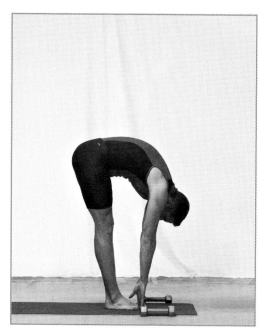

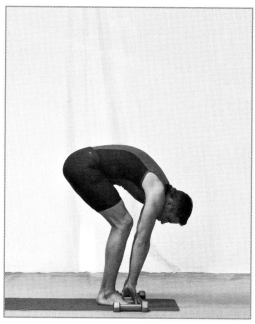

3. Standing Forward Bend

Exhale and dive forward and down. Fold your torso over your thighs, lower your forehead toward your knees or shins, and reach your fingertips to the mat by the sides of your toes.

4. Transition

Inhale to prepare for Plank pose by softly bending your knees and lifting your head up.

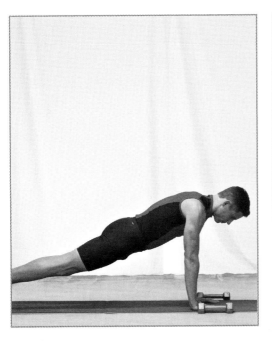
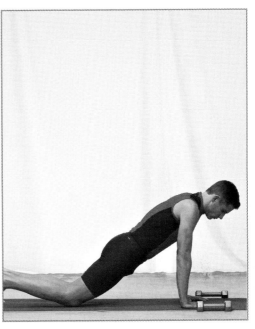

5. Plank (High Pushup)

Exhale and either jump both legs back or step back one leg at a time. Curl your toes into the mat, pressing your heels back with your feet hip-width apart. Align your hands under your shoulders, with your fingers spread wide, and release your shoulders down and back away from your ears. Create one straight line of energy from the crown of your head to your heels, with your arms and legs straight, hips even, back flat, head neutral, and gaze slightly forward. Activate your lower back, glutes, and legs. Engage your core. This is an excellent pose to develop strength in your shoulders, arms, chest, and abdominal region.

Modification:

Lower softly to your knees, keeping your arms straight.

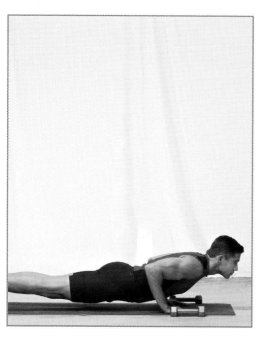

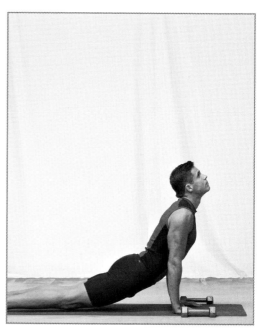

6. Chaturanga (Low Pushup)

From Plank pose, inhale to prepare, and as you exhale, bend your elbows to lower your body 2 to 3 inches from the mat. Press your elbows into the sides of your torso and keep your shoulders down and back away from your ears. Shift your head and upper body slightly forward, so your elbows are at the midpoint of your torso and your upper arms are parallel to the mat. Keep your legs straight and active with your heels pressing back. Engage your core. Maintain a flat back and long spine with a straight line of energy from the crown of your head to your heels. Lift your head slightly and gaze forward. This pose requires tremendous strength and works every muscle group in your body.

Modification:

Lower softly to your knees. Keep your elbows bent and your torso 2 to 3 inches off the mat. (See photo inset on page 84.)

7. Upward-Facing Dog

From Chaturanga pose, inhale and press the tops of your feet into the mat and straighten your arms, keeping your wrists under your shoulders while you lift up your chest and head. Open your shoulders wide and arch your lower back. Release your shoulders down and back away from your ears. Engage your lower back and core while activating your glutes and legs.

Modification:

Keep your legs on the mat and softly bend your elbows. (See photo inset on page 85.)

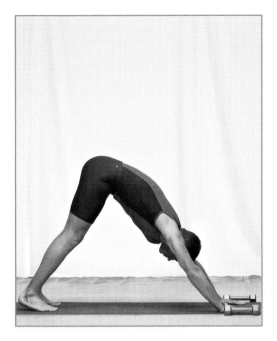

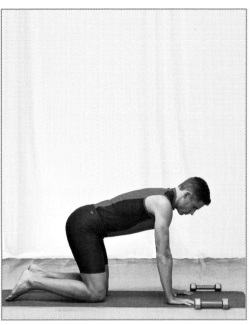

8. Downward-Facing Dog

From Upward-Facing Dog, exhale and lift your tailbone high to create an inverted "V" with your body. Press your armpits toward your knees, your chest toward your thighs, and your heels down to the mat. Keep your head neutral and your back flat, with your spine long. Keep your arms and legs straight and active. Make sure your feet are hip-width apart, with your toes spread wide. Check your hands to make sure they are shoulder-width apart, with your fingers spread wide. Rotate your inner elbows toward each other to open your shoulders and improve your flexibility and range of motion. Press into the knuckles of your index fingers to relieve any strain that may develop in your hands, wrists, and forearms. Feel a straight line of energy from your tailbone to your fingertips and your tailbone to your heels. Downward-Facing Dog is one of the few yoga poses that increases strength of the entire body while at the same time stretching and relaxing the entire body. Hold for 4 breaths.

9. Transition

From Downward-Facing Dog, lower your knees to the mat under your hips, coming to all fours, with your hands under your shoulders, your back flat, and your head neutral.

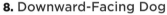

CHAPTER 7

F L O O R
P O S E S

The focus for the poses in this chapter is on flexibility, though I have added some poses that strengthen your arms, legs, abs, and lower back. In Bird Dog/Flying Airplane and Boat poses, you add more resistance by using the dumbbells. If you're just starting out, put the dumbbells on the side and just focus on the movement itself. I recommend that you hold most of these poses for a minimum of 4 breaths.

BIRD DOG/FLYING AIRPLANE

This pose helps to strengthen and stretch your entire back and spinal column. You'll also strengthen your arms, shoulders, abs, glutes, and thighs.

1. Prepare

Come to all fours with your hands under your shoulders, your knees under your hips, the tops of your feet pressing into the mat, and your toes pointing back. Take hold of one dumbbell in your left hand. Extend the left dumbbell straight forward, resting the bottom dumbbell head on the mat, with your left palm facing right. Gaze toward the mat, keeping your head neutral and your back flat. Press your right hand firmly into the mat, spreading your fingers wide.

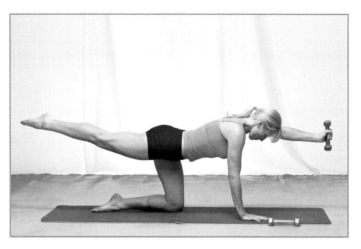

2. Start Position

Inhale and, at the same time, lift your right foot and the left dumbbell off the mat. Extend your right leg straight back in line with your right hip, pointing your toes, and the left dumbbell straight forward in line with your shoulder. It should feel like someone is pulling back on your right foot and forward on your left hand. Engage your core.

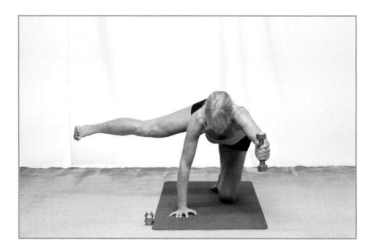

3. Exhale and flex your right foot to activate your right leg. Inhale and extend your right leg straight out to your right side, perpendicular to and in line with your right hip. Exhale and return to the start position (#2).

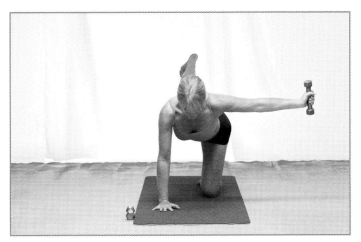

4. Inhale and extend the left dumbbell straight out to your left side, perpendicular to and in line with your left shoulder. Exhale and return to the start position (#2).

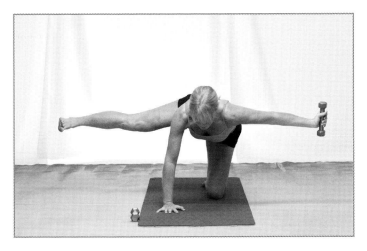

5. Static Contraction
Inhale and repeat #3 and #4 with both your right leg and the left dumbbell together. Hold the movement at peak contraction. Exhale and then inhale to enhance the peak contraction. Exhale and return to the start position (#2).

6. Repeat #2 to #5 with your left leg and with the dumbbell in your right hand.

COW/CAT

This is a great stretch for relieving tension and stress in your lower back. The deep abdominal breathing in this pose will create relaxation throughout the body.

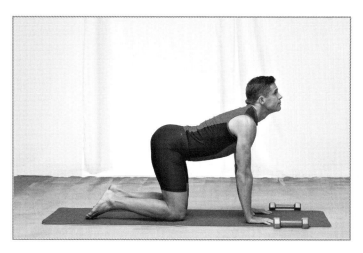

1. Cow

From Bird Dog/Flying Airplane pose, release the right dumbbell to the mat. Place your hands under your shoulders and keep your knees under your hips, with the tops of your feet pressing into the mat and your toes pointing back. Create a straight line of energy from the crown of your head to your tailbone. Place your head in a neutral position and gaze at a point on the mat, relaxing your neck and shoulders. Inhale and slowly lift your head and gaze up while arching your lower back.

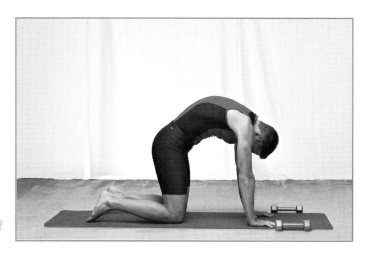

2. Cat

Exhale and slowly lower your head, tucking your chin to your chest. Release your tailbone down, while rounding your upper back and shoulders. Draw your navel up and in toward your spine. Hold for 4 breaths, while inhaling into Cow and exhaling into Cat.

PIGEON

This is one of the best poses to open tight hips. You'll feel a deep stretch in your glutes, hip flexors, and inner thighs—perfect after running, cycling, or any cardio activity.

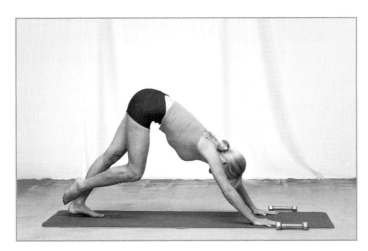

1. From Cat pose, come to a neutral position on all fours and curl your toes into the mat. Inhale to prepare, exhale, and press your tailbone to the ceiling, and your heels down to the mat (Downward-Facing Dog). Place the top of your right foot on the back of your left heel. Keep your left leg straight and active, getting a great stretch for the back of your left leg.

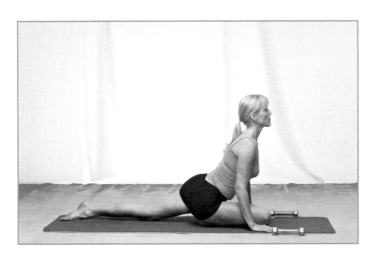

2. Inhale to prepare, exhale, and bring your right knee up to your right palm, placing your right foot to the left side of the mat. Lower your left knee to the mat and walk the top of your left foot back, keeping your left leg straight. Inhale and arch your lower back, open your shoulders wide, and lift up your chest. Tilt your head back and gaze up. Keep your elbows soft and release your shoulders down and back away from your ears. Hold for 4 breaths.

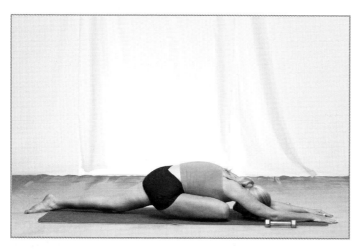

3. Inhale to prepare, exhale, lower your elbows and forearms to the mat, and walk your hands forward, keeping your arms straight. Fold your torso forward and tuck your chin to your chest, lowering your forehead to the mat. Keep your hips square and press your right glute and your left hip flexor down toward the mat. So much power is derived in this area; use your breath to release it. Hold for 4 breaths.

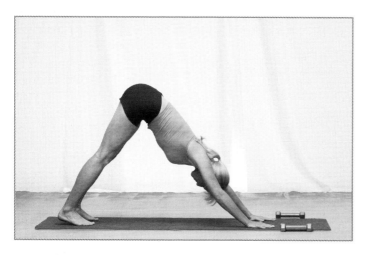

4. Inhale and walk your hands back in line with your shoulders and curl your left toes into the mat. Exhale and press back into Downward-Facing Dog pose.

5. Repeat #1 to #4 with the opposite leg.

FOREARM PLANK

This is an excellent pose to strengthen your triceps, chest, shoulders, and abdominal region. It's a great way to improve your strength for Chaturanga and Upward-Facing Dog poses.

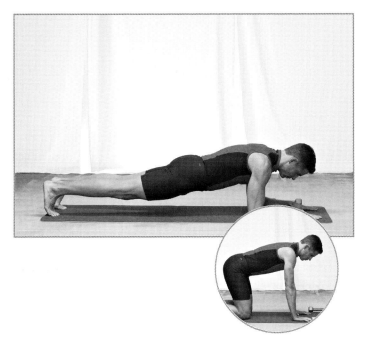

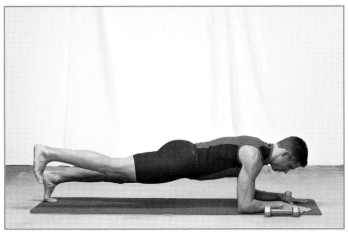

1. From Downward-Facing Dog pose, inhale to prepare, exhale, and lower your knees to the mat under your hips (see inset). Lower your elbows to the mat under your shoulders, with your forearms extended straight forward and your palms pressing into the mat, shoulder-width apart. Spread your fingers wide. Extend your right and left legs straight back on your toes, with your feet hip-width apart. Create one straight line of energy from the crown of your head to your heels. Keep your head neutral, your back flat, your legs active, and your shoulders down and back away from your ears. Engage your core. Hold for 4 breaths.

2. Inhale and raise your right foot 1 inch off the mat, flexing your right foot and pressing your right heel back. Hold for 2 breaths. Exhale and lower your right foot to the mat.

3. Repeat #2 with your left foot.

LOCUST

Locust pose stretches and strengthens your lower back. Not only does it help to relieve lower back pain, but the massaging effect on your stomach can help stimulate digestion.

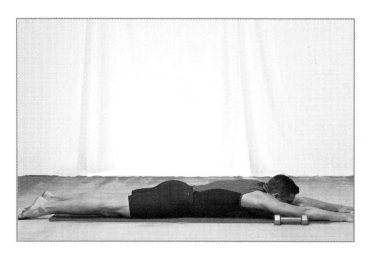

1. From Forearm Plank pose, lie face down on the mat, with your arms and legs fully extended, your palms facing downward, and the tops of your feet flat, toes pointing back.

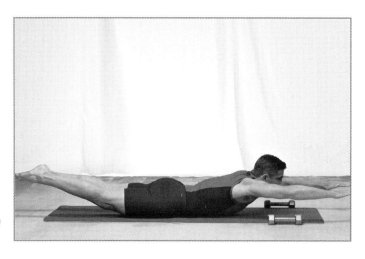

2. Inhale to prepare, exhale, and use the strength of your lower back to lift your chin, chest, arms, and legs off the mat. Feel your fingertips reaching forward and your toes reaching back. Hold for 2 breaths.

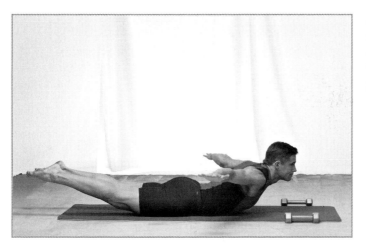

3. Bring your arms straight out to your sides, with your palms facing the mat. Inhale to prepare, exhale, and lift your chin, chest, arms, and legs higher. Hold for 2 breaths.

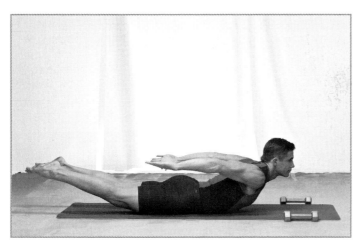

4. Bring your arms back, with your palms facing upward. Inhale to prepare, exhale, and lift higher. Hold for 2 breaths. On the last exhalation, return your chin, chest, arms, and legs to the mat.

BOW

This pose will give you a great stretch in your quads, hip flexors, lower back, and shoulders. If you have any history of lower back pain or injury, you may want to skip this pose. You can also try doing this one leg at a time.

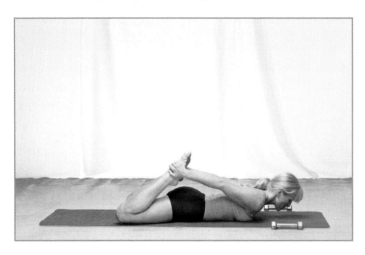

1. From Locust pose, bend your knees and take hold of the tops of your feet or ankles. Open your knees a little wider than hip-width apart.

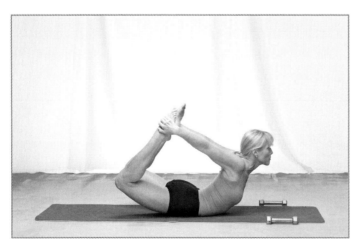

2. Inhale to prepare, exhale, and press the tops of your feet or ankles into your hands, lifting your shoulders, chest, knees, and thighs off the mat. Squeeze your shoulder blades together and open your chest and shoulders wide. Hold for 4 breaths.

REST

The goal for this pose is to relax your full body, so you feel completely centered and at ease. Allow all of your tension and stress to flow from your body into the mat.

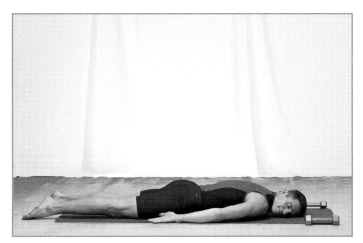

From Bow pose, release your ankles, let your legs lower softly to the mat, and place your arms to your sides, with your palms facing upward. Turn your head to the left side, resting gently on your right ear, and softly close your eyes. Hold for 4 breaths. Turn your head to the right side, resting gently on your left ear. Hold for 4 breaths. Focus on total relaxation. Connect with your breath, feeling it deep, full, and long. Your body will begin to feel centered, creating balance, equilibrium, and relaxation.

HALF BOAT/FULL BOAT

This pose is named Boat because your body resembles a boat with your arms as the oars. Boat pose is a challenging pose, great for strengthening and toning your abs.

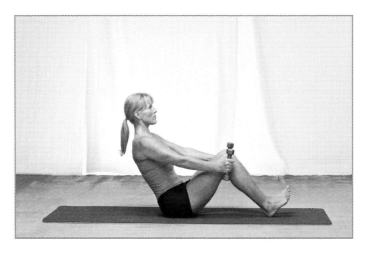

1. Prepare

From Rest pose, roll over and come to a seated position on the mat. Bend your knees with your heels on the mat and your toes pointing upward. Take hold of a dumbbell in each hand and extend the dumbbells to the sides of your knees, with your arms straight. Keep your back flat and release your shoulders down and back away from your ears.

Modification:

If you're having trouble keeping your back flat and holding the pose, don't use the dumbbells in this sequence.

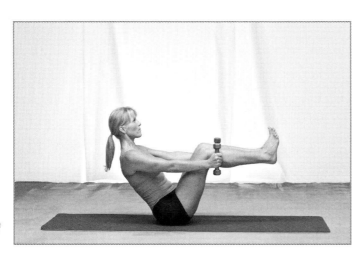

2. Half Boat

Inhale and lift your right foot off the mat and then bring your left foot to meet it. Flex both feet and keep your lower legs parallel to the mat. Gaze over your toes. Hold for 2 breaths.

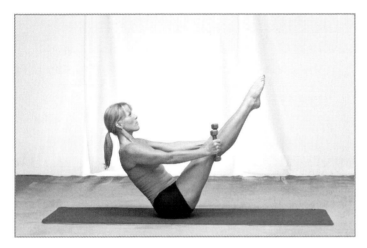

3. Full Boat

Inhale to prepare, exhale, and straighten your legs upward. Use the strength of your abs to keep your torso from leaning backward. Point your toes and activate your quads. If this pose is too challenging, remain in Half Boat instead. Hold for 4 breaths.

OBLIQUE CRUNCH

Strong abs and obliques are important for posture and for preventing back injury. This is one of the best poses for strengthening and toning your entire core region.

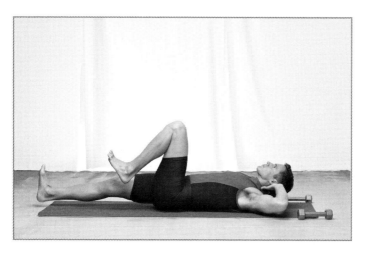

1. From Boat pose, lower the dumbbells to the mat. Take hold of the backs of your thighs and gently lower your torso down one vertebra at a time to the mat. Softly cradle your head with your hands and spread your elbows wide. Extend your right leg straight forward 1 inch off the mat and bend your left leg so that your left thigh is perpendicular to the mat. Lift your shoulder blades 1 inch off the mat. Flex both of your feet. The muscles in your right leg should be active and strong.

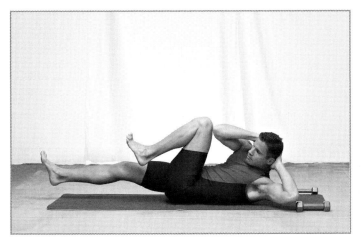

2. Engage your left oblique, inhale to prepare, exhale, and lift your right elbow to the outside of your left knee. Keep your left elbow back. Hold for 4 breaths.

3. Repeat #1 and #2 with your left leg forward and your left elbow reaching to the outside of your right knee.

CHAPTER 8

COOLDOWN

The Cooldown is a very important part of the Iron Yoga practice. Here you will allow your body to relax and let your mind ease. These poses really allow you to connect with your breath, so you should focus on your breathing first and foremost. The final pose, Hero pose, is a complete relaxation and meditation pose. Let all the tension you released through your Iron Yoga practice melt from your body. Stay in this pose as long as you like. Several minutes are ideal for meditation.

RECLINED TWIST

Twists like this one are great for massaging your digestive organs. This pose also helps you release tension in your lower back.

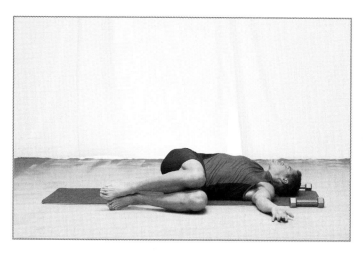

1. From Oblique Crunch pose, bring your knees to-gether and extend your arms out to the sides with your palms facing upward. Let your knees fall to your left side with your right knee on top of your left knee. Softly turn your head to the right side. Hold for 2 breaths. This is a great stretch for your lower back and hip area.

2. Repeat #1 on the opposite side.

SEATED FORWARD BEND

This is a great stretch for the back of your legs and lower back. You may not be able to touch your toes at first, but go as far as you can without feeling pain and overstretching your muscles.

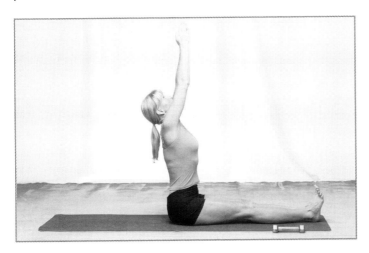

1. From Reclined Twist pose, take hold of the backs of your thighs and gently lift your torso up off the mat one vertebra at a time. Extend both of your legs straight forward with the backs of your legs pressing firmly into the mat. Flex your feet and activate your legs. Inhale and raise your arms straight out to the sides and high overhead, pressing together your palms and gazing over your fingertips.

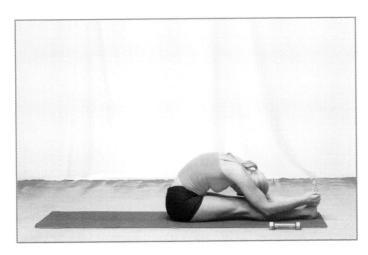

2. Exhale and lower your arms straight forward, palms facing downward, and reach long for your shins, ankles, feet, and toes. Fold your torso over your thighs, tuck your chin to your chest, lower your forehead to your knees or shins, and release your shoulders down and back away from your ears. Hold for 4 breaths. Inhale and release your toes, walk your fingertips slowly up the fronts of your legs, and straighten your torso.

BOUND ANGLE

This is an excellent pose for releasing tightness in the groin area and opening the hips. Make sure not to force your knees down to the floor but to let your groin open naturally.

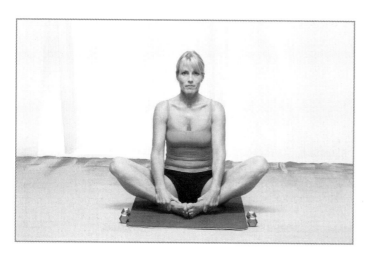

1. From Seated Forward Bend pose , sit up firmly on your sit bones, bend your knees, and take hold of the tops of your feet. Place the soles of your feet together in front of your groin area and release your shoulders down and back away from your ears.

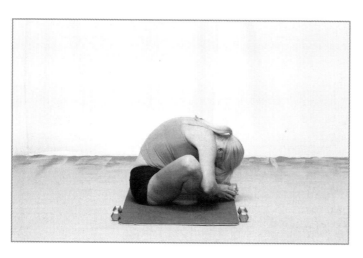

2. Inhale to prepare, exhale and bend your torso forward, and lower your forehead toward your ankles and feet. Tuck your chin to your chest. Hold for 4 breaths.

SEATED ONE-LEGGED EXTENSION

The bent leg in this stretch helps to open your hip while stretching your inner thigh and groin area. You will feel a great stretch in your hamstring and calf of your straight leg, while alleviating any tightness in your lower back.

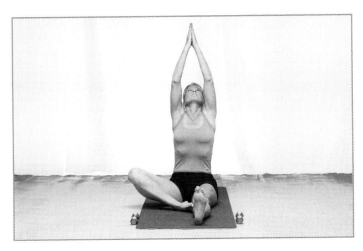

1. From Bound Angle pose, extend your left leg straight forward. Flex your left foot and activate your left leg. Bend your right knee and place the sole of your right foot on the inside of your left upper thigh. Try to keep your right knee out wide and low to the mat. Inhale and raise your arms straight out to the sides and high overhead, pressing together your palms and gazing over your fingertips.

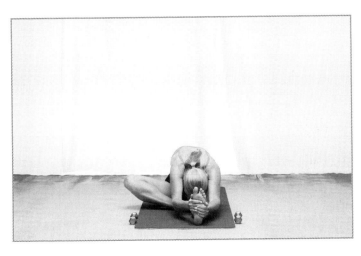

2. Exhale and lower your arms straight forward, palms facing downward, and reach long for your left shin, ankle, foot, and toes. Fold your torso over your left thigh, tuck your chin to your chest, lower your forehead to your left knee or shin, and release your shoulders down and back away from your ears. Hold for 4 breaths. Inhale and release your left toes, walk your fingertips slowly up the front of your left leg, and straighten your torso.

3. Repeat #1 and #2 on the opposite side.

SEATED ONE-LEGGED TWIST

This is a great stretch for the iliotibial band—the thick, wide band of tissue starting at the hip and running down the outer portion of the leg to just below the knee. The twisting movement tones the waist and increases flexibility in your lower back and hip joint.

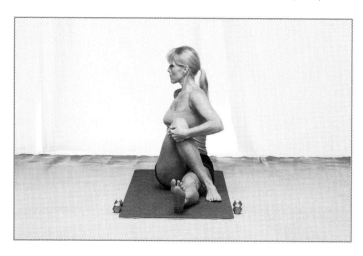

1. From Seated One-Legged Extension pose, bend your right knee, cross your right foot over your left leg, and press your right foot firmly into the mat outside your left knee. Place your left palm on the outside of your right knee and plant your right palm on the mat about 4 inches behind your right buttock. Inhale to prepare, then exhale and twist your torso and head to the right side while pressing your right knee gently toward your left shoulder. Gaze over your right shoulder. Hold for 4 breaths.

2. Repeat #1 on the opposite side.

SEATED WIDE-ANGLE SEQUENCE

This series of stretches gives you a deep and intense stretch for your hamstrings, groin area, and lower back. Spread your legs only as far as you can without feeling discomfort. If you can't touch your toes, that's fine—just go as deep as you can and ease comfortably into the stretch.

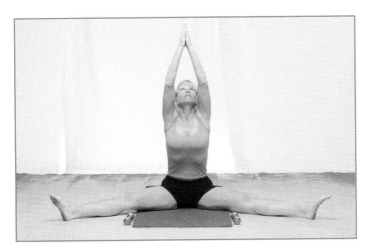

1. From Seated One-Legged Twist pose, sit up tall, firmly on your sit bones, and extend your legs straight out to the sides. Point your toes and activate your legs. Inhale and raise your arms straight out to the sides and high overhead, pressing together your palms and gazing over your fingertips.

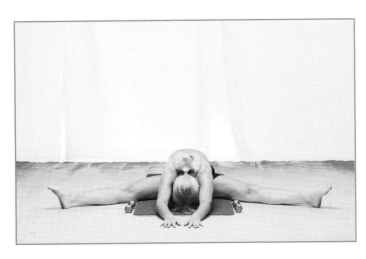

2. Exhale and lower your arms straight forward, palms facing downward, as you reach long on the mat in front of you. Fold your torso forward, lengthening your spine and keeping your back flat. Tuck your chin to your chest, lower your forehead to the mat, and release your shoulders down and back away from your ears. Hold for 4 breaths.

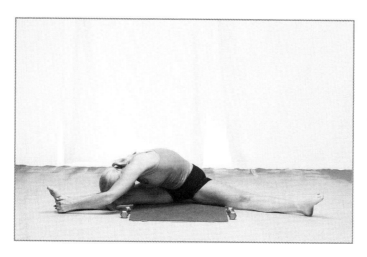

3. Inhale and walk your fingertips over to your right foot. Exhale and fold your torso over your right thigh and lower your forehead to your right knee or shin. Hold for 4 breaths.

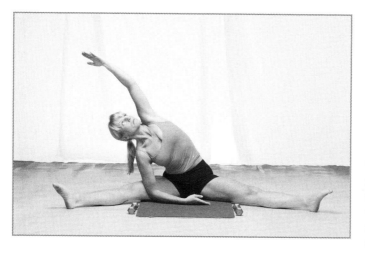

4. Inhale and walk your fingertips up the front of your right leg. Exhale and place your right elbow on the mat inside your right knee. Inhale and raise your left arm overhead and to the right side. Exhale and contract your right oblique, leaning your torso to the right side. Turn your head up to the left and gaze over your left fingertips. Hold for 4 breaths. On the last exhalation, fold your torso over your left thigh.

5. Repeat #3 and #4 on your opposite side and then sit up tall.

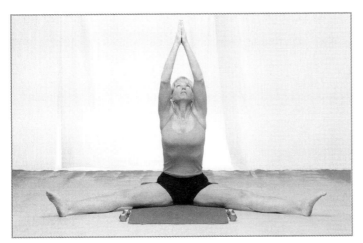

6. Repeat #1.

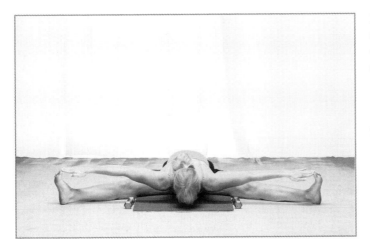

7. Exhale and lower your arms straight to the sides and reach long for your shins, ankles, feet, and toes. Fold your torso forward, lengthening your spine and keeping your back flat. Tuck your chin to your chest, lower your forehead to the mat, and release your shoulders down and back away from your ears. Hold for 4 breaths.

SEATED CROSS-LEGGED SEQUENCE

This is the final series of stretches in the Cooldown. If you have trouble keeping your knees level with your hips, try sitting on the edge of a cushion or folded-up towel.

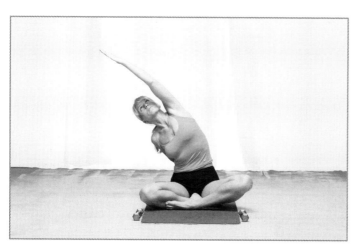

1. From Seated Wide-Angle Sequence, come to a comfortable cross-legged position. Place your right palm on the mat about 4 inches behind your right buttock. Inhale and raise your left arm straight overhead. Exhale and contract your right oblique, leaning your torso to the right side. Turn your head up to the left and gaze over your left fingertips. Hold for 4 breaths. Repeat on your opposite side.

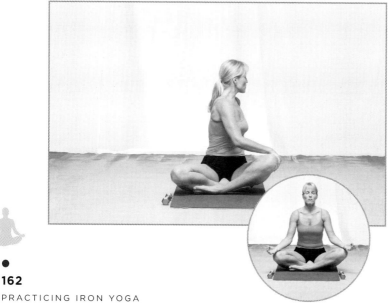

2. Place your left palm on the mat about 4 inches behind your left buttock and your right palm on the outside of your left knee. Inhale to prepare, then exhale and twist your torso and head to the left side. Gaze over your left shoulder. Hold for 4 breaths. Repeat on your opposite side.

3. Place the tops of your hands on each knee and gently press together your thumb and index finger. Release your shoulders down and back away from your ears. Softly close your eyes. Hold for 4 breaths.

CHILD'S POSE

This pose releases all the tension in your shoulders and neck and brings circulation to the lower back and abs.

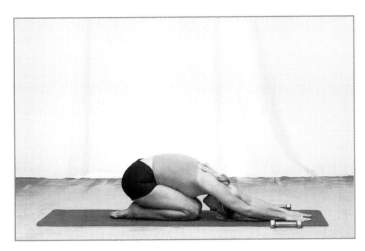

1. From Seated Cross-Legged Sequence, turn over onto all fours, place your knees together and heels slightly apart with your hands under your shoulders and your knees under your hips. Sit back into your heels with the tops of your feet pressing into the mat and toes pointing back. Walk your hands and arms straight forward and fold your torso over your thighs. Tuck your chin to your chest, release your shoulders down and back away from your ears, and lower your forehead to the mat. Focus on complete rest and relaxation for your mind and body. Hold for 4 breaths.

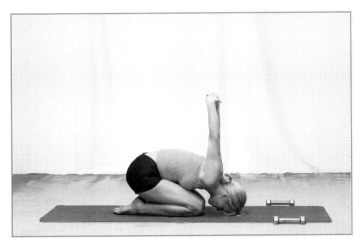

2. Place your hands together over your tailbone, interlocking your fingertips. Inhale to prepare, exhale and lift your hands and arms up, and gently pull back, getting a good final stretch for your triceps, rear delts, and upper back. Hold for 2 breaths.

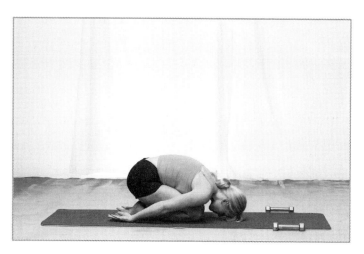

3. Lower your hands to your tailbone. Separate your hands and place the tops of your hands on the mat by the sides of your toes, palms facing upward. Make sure to keep your shoulders relaxed. Sit back deeper and extend your torso farther. Hold for 4 breaths.

HERO

This is your final cooldown pose in Iron Yoga. Take as much time as you need here to relax and enjoy the accomplishment of completing your Iron Yoga practice.

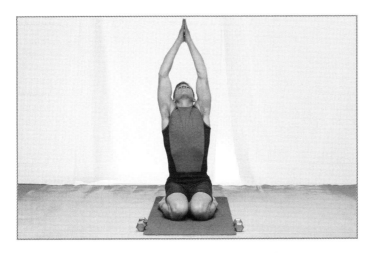

1. From Child's pose, gently and slowly lift your torso off your thighs, coming up one vertebra at a time. Sit back into your heels and ankles and round your shoulders up, back, and down.

2. Inhale and raise your arms straight out to the sides and high overhead, your palms pressing together and gazing over your fingertips.

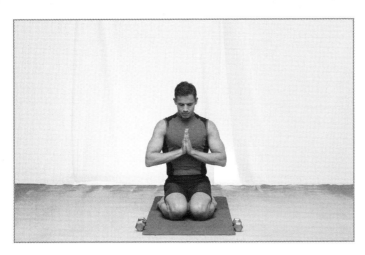

3. Exhale and release your arms down to your sides and place your palms together over your heart. Softly close your eyes and bow your head into your hands. Connect one last time with breath. Feel and hear your breath. Use the breath to ease your mind, open your heart, and cleanse your soul. Let your breath heal, rejuvenate, and reenergize your body.

IRON YOGA
FOR SPORTS

As an athlete, you will find that Iron Yoga can be complementary to your sport and even help you improve your performance. Practicing Iron Yoga a few times a week can help you stay flexible and strong. The Iron Yoga practice is designed to strengthen your muscles but not add bulk to them. As an athlete, it is important to have long, lean muscles that are explosive and don't restrict range of motion.

The Iron Yoga practice helps to keep your muscles and joints active. During an intense training workout like a 10k run or 50-mile bike ride, your muscles must work hard. As you push through those final miles, your muscles sometimes go into overdrive and fill with lactic acid, a waste product of intense muscle activity and fatigue. The Iron Yoga workout prepares the body and mind for these moments of lactic acid buildup. The intensity of the Iron Yoga practice will create the same muscle burn feeling in the legs that is commonly felt during a training workout or competition.

Perhaps one of the most important ways Iron Yoga can enhance your sports performance is by improving your breath awareness. One of the best ways to do this is to simply breathe more fully. The deep abdominal breathing techniques you've been practicing in Iron Yoga can help you achieve this. By stretching all the respiratory muscles in your lungs, you can actually increase your lung capacity. As you apply the deep abdominal breathing to your favorite sport, you'll find that you will achieve a more intense and focused workout.

What about the anxiety and stress of competition? If you're a runner, you know all too well about the pre-race jitters that can sap your focus and energy. That's not to say a little anxiety is all bad. Those pre-race jitters can provide some adrenaline to push your body and stimulate your focus. However, excess anxiety can hurt your performance. The yogic breathing you've practiced in Iron Yoga can help you ease some of that excess anxiety and transform it into a competitive edge.

So whatever sport or fitness activity you enjoy, Iron Yoga can help you stay healthy for a lifetime of fitness. For each sport I've included some basic health benefits, as well as common problems—and an Iron Yoga fix.

RUNNING

Running is one of the best ways to improve your cardio conditioning. It's also a great way to burn calories and lose fat. Running races, whether a 5k or a marathon, is the perfect motivation to keep you in shape.

COMMON PROBLEMS

Unfortunately, running puts extreme stress on your body. Due to the constant contraction and repetitive motion, the knee and ankle joint are particularly prone to injury. Muscles in the lower back, hips, and legs tend to tighten and shorten, also leading to injury.

IRON YOGA FIX

You should focus on stretching your legs and lower body as thoroughly as possible. This includes the quads, hamstrings, and calves. Downward-Facing Dog is a great way to stretch the backs of your leg muscles and lower back. Pigeon can help to keep your hips open and flexible. Dancer's stretches your quads and hip flexors. The upper-body Iron Yoga strength movements help keep your shoulders, arms, chest, and back strong. Triangle; balancing poses such as Tree, Warrior 3, Standing Leg Raise, and Eagle; and the Power Lunge Sequence all help you develop tremendous leg strength and muscular endurance.

CYCLING

Whether you're on the open road or indoors in a group spinning class, cycling provides a terrific cardio workout. Not only is it a great way to control your weight and strengthen your legs, but it puts a lot less stress on your joints than running.

If your bike is not fitted properly, the repetitive motion of cycling can cause your knee and Achilles tendon to become inflamed, and you can also put undue pressure on your back. Always make sure your bike seat is adjusted to the proper height to protect your knees and hip joints. Leaning on the handlebars can also cause your wrist joints to become inflamed.

IRON YOGA FIX

Stretch and strengthen your lower body, paying close attention to your quads, hamstrings, and hips. Standing Forward Bend is a great lower-body stretch for the hamstrings. Keeping your back strong and flexible is also important to counterbalance the "hunched over" position of your body on the bike. The Lat Pulldown and Row movements help to strengthen your back muscles. Bow, Cow/Cat, and Downward-Facing Dog help to stretch your back. The Wrist Curl movements are ideal for strengthening the muscles that help you grip the handlebars. All of the leg-balancing poses build muscular endurance in your legs for those extra-long rides and will make the pedal stroke symmetrical. The Power Lunge Sequence strengthens your legs, which will enable you to generate more power and apply more force to the pedal stroke.

SWIMMING

Swimming provides an unbelievable cardio workout with little stress on your joints. It's a perfect cross-training sport when you want to take some time off from running or cycling.

COMMON PROBLEMS

Most swimming-related injuries involve the shoulder. Your rotator cuff can become inflamed by fatigue and overuse, while your shoulder can become inflexible. Poor balance in the water causes your legs to sink and creates unnecessary drag. If you're not used to rhythmic deep abdominal breathing, your stamina and performance in the pool can also suffer.

IRON YOGA FIX

The External/Internal Rotation movements help to strengthen your rotator cuffs. The improved balance you learn on land will carry over to better balance and a better feel in the water. The weight-training exercises for the back and triceps will strengthen the pull phase of the swim stroke. Half Moon and Standing Leg Raise will help streamline your position in the water. The core-strengthening poses and exercises will improve body rotation to generate more power and propulsion. And Hero is great for improving flexibility in the ankles to make your kick stronger.

TENNIS (AND OTHER RACQUET SPORTS)

Tennis and other racquet sports like racquetball, squash, and badminton are a fun way to build up your strength, cardio, balance, and agility. The competitive aspect of these sports can also keep you motivated so you don't feel like you're working out at all.

COMMON PROBLEMS

For these racquet sports, the biggest problem comes from overuse of the elbow, shoulder, and knees. You're probably familiar with the term *tennis elbow*. This condition involves inflammation of the muscles and tendons along the outside of the forearm. In terms of the lower body, quick movements around the court can cause knee and foot injuries.

IRON YOGA FIX

All of the balancing poses are particularly helpful in improving your balance and coordination as you react and move quickly across the court. For your shoulder and rotator cuff, the External/Internal Rotation is a great strength builder and will also improve your shoulder flexibility and range of motion. The Sun Salutation and Wrist Curl and Reverse Wrist Curl exercises will build your wrists and forearms and strengthen your grip.

GOLF

While golf may not give you the heart-pumping cardio workout you'd get from running or swimming, it does place its own physical and mental demands on your body, including the need for a sharp mental focus and concentration.

COMMON PROBLEMS

The extreme twisting motion of the golf swing can strain your back and obliques. The muscles on the opposite side of your dominant arm may be particularly vulnerable. Like tennis elbow, *golfer's elbow* is an inflammation of the muscles and tendons along the forearm, but in this case, along the *inside* of the forearm.

Breathing and balancing poses help to improve your focus and concentration. Oblique Twist and Half Moon are great for strengthening your sides, while the Standing Back Bend gives your back a good stretch, too. Wrist Curls and Reverse Wrist Curls help to give you strong forearms and wrists for a powerful swing. To release the tension in your torso from the swinging motion, you can try the Seated Cross-Legged Sequence, Dancer's, and Triangle.

SKIING (CROSS-COUNTRY AND DOWNHILL)

Both cross-country and downhill skiing work every major muscle group in your body. You can get a great cardio workout with little stress to your joints.

COMMON PROBLEMS

While cross-country skiing is relatively risk-free, downhill skiing is more risky. You're going to need quick reflexes and flexible muscles to maneuver through the constant twists and turns. You're also going to need strong back and leg muscles to hold your body in a bent-knee position and protect yourself from a fall. One of the most common injury areas is the knee—which is particularly vulnerable to ligament tears of the ACL (anterior cruciate ligament). Broken or sprained lower-body joints are also common.

IRON YOGA FIX

Chair simulates the body position in downhill skiing. Holding this pose for a minute or two is a great way to build muscular endurance in your legs and lower back. If you have tight hips, Pigeon helps to open your hip flexors. All of the balancing poses will help to improve your balance and coordination on steep slopes and to prevent falls.

INLINE SKATING

Inline skating is another great cardio sport with little impact on your joints. Coordination and agility are crucial to maintaining the fluid gliding motion needed for skating.

COMMON PROBLEMS

The main problems from inline skating are falling and twisting. Your wrists are particularly vulnerable during a fall. Your leg joints from your hips to your ankles can also take a hit from a twist in the wrong direction.

IRON YOGA FIX

Balancing poses help build agility and coordination to prevent falls. Strong abs also help you stay balanced, so try focusing on Boat and Oblique Crunch. If you do fall forward onto your hands, the Sun Salutations help develop your wrist and forearm strength to protect your wrists. For strong and flexible leg muscles, the Power Lunge Sequence gives your lower body a complete workout.

ROWING

Whether you're on the water in a canoe or kayak or in the gym on a rowing machine, rowing is a great way to strengthen your upper body. What's more, you'll get an intense cardio and fat-burning workout.

COMMON PROBLEMS

Because it involves little or no stress on your legs, the majority of problems caused by rowing stem from the repetitive motion of the rowing movement. Impacted most are your back, shoulders, elbows, and wrists.

IRON YOGA FIX

To build your back muscles, the Row and Lat Pulldown poses are beneficial. Chair is also a great way to build up your back as well as your legs. For strong wrists and forearms, focus on the Wrist Curl and Reverse Wrist Curl. Cow/Cat is a great way to relieve some of the stress on your back caused by rowing. The Sun Salutations will help to release tension in your entire body and counteract the hunched-over rowing position.

IRON YOGA
AT A GLANCE

In this section, you'll find a quick reference to all of the Iron Yoga sequences in the book. With these photos you'll be able to see the flow from one pose to the next. Bear in mind that you'll still need to refer back to the text to incorporate the static contractions, correct number of repetitions, and breathing cues. Nonetheless, these at-a-glance photos can greatly enhance your overall understanding of the Iron Yoga workout.

WARMUP SEQUENCE

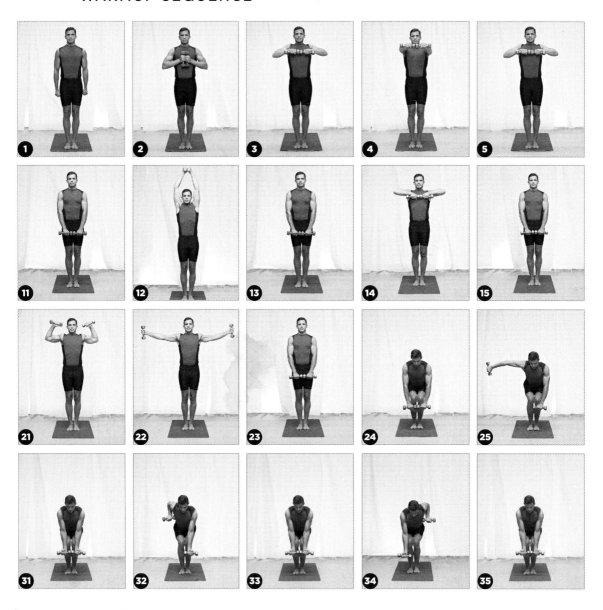

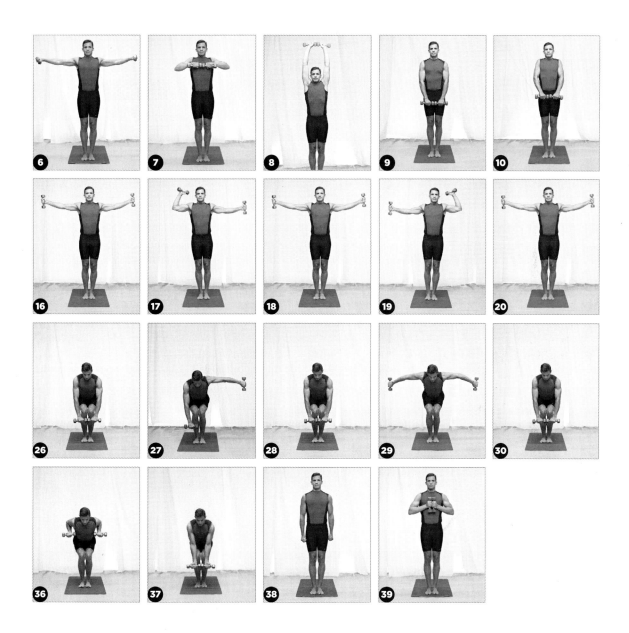

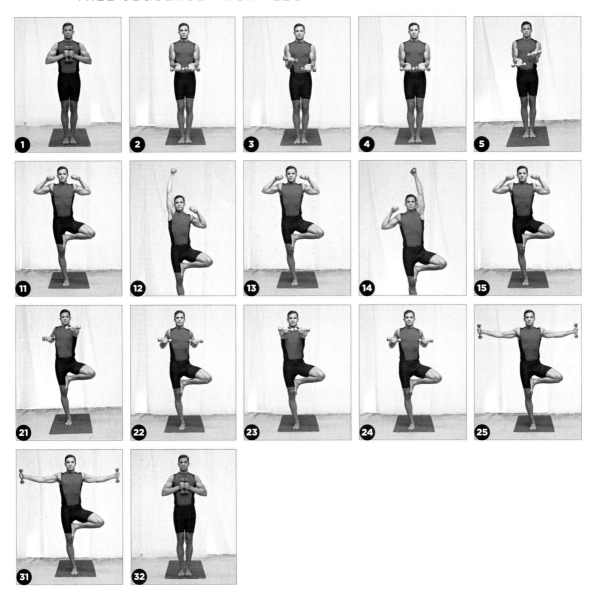

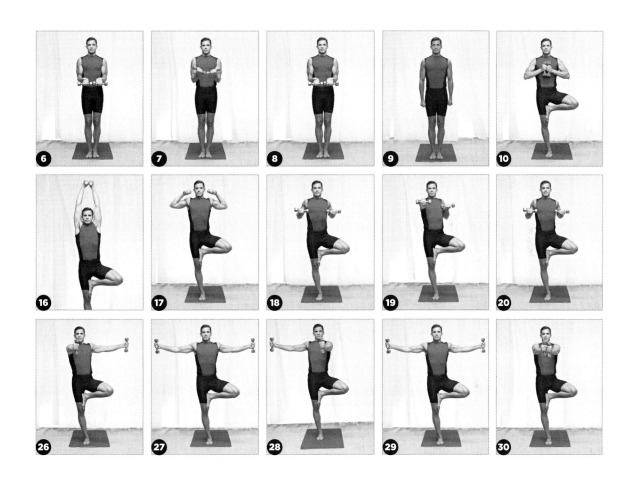

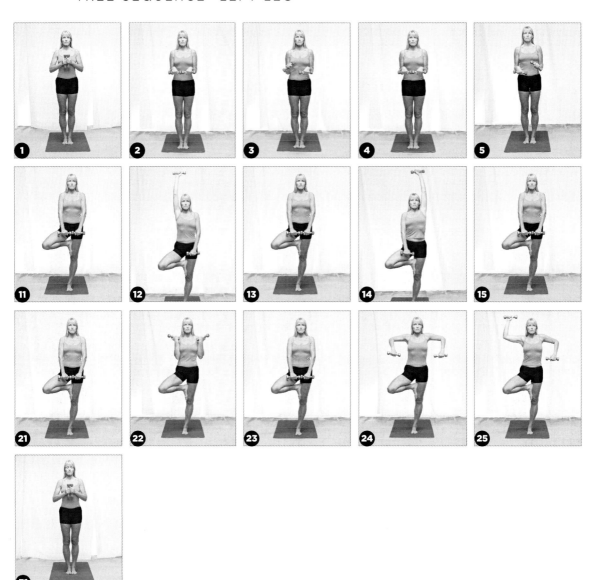

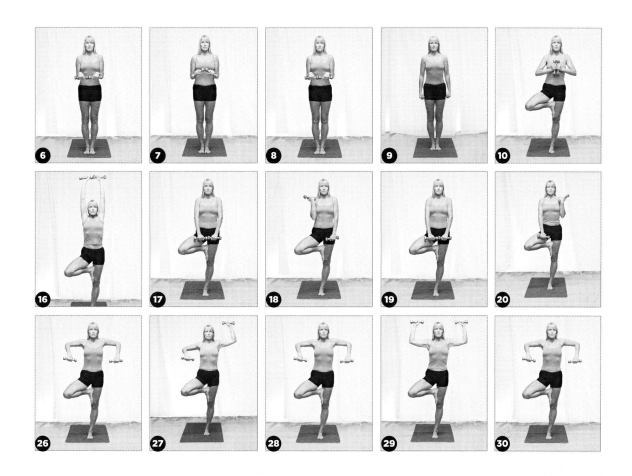

POWER LUNGE SEQUENCE—RIGHT LEG

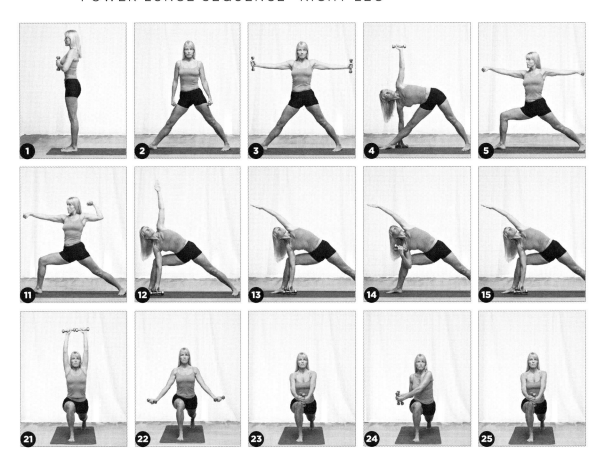

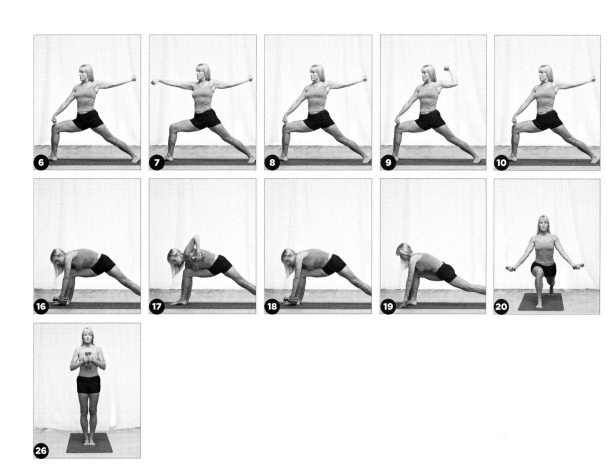

SUN SALUTATION—SEQUENCE I

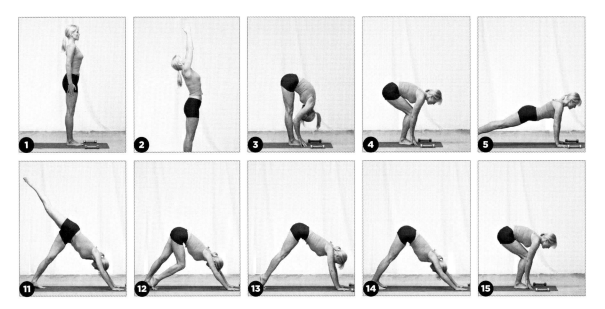

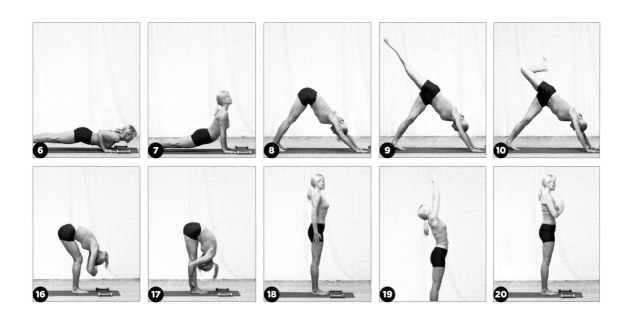

POWER LUNGE SEQUENCE—LEFT LEG

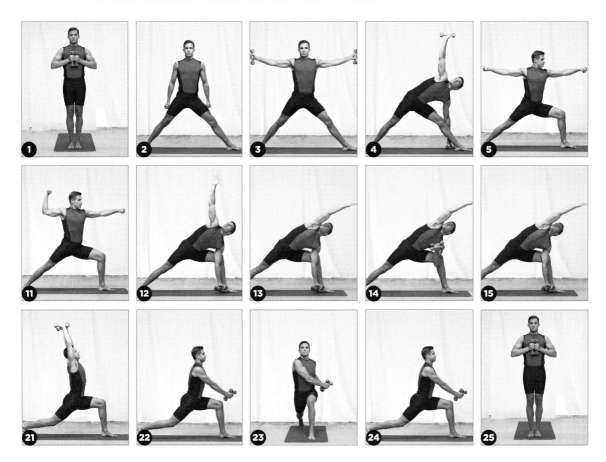

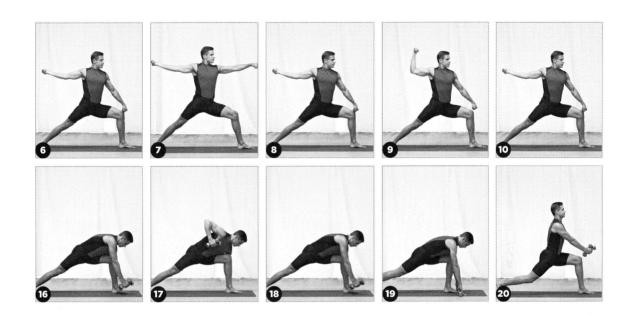

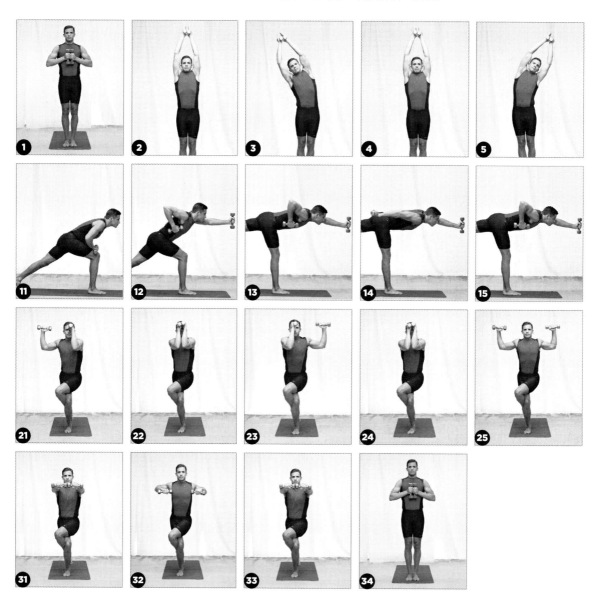

SEATED CROSS-LEGGED SEQUENCE

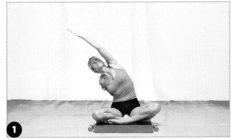

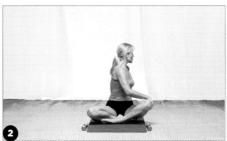

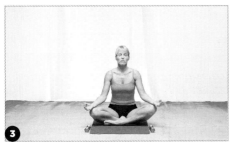

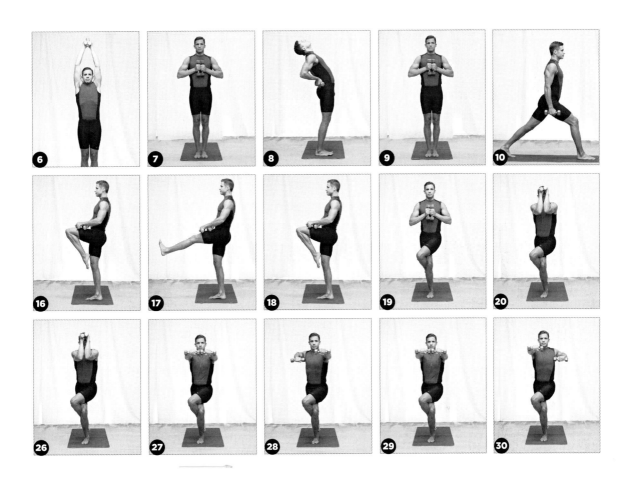

IRON YOGA AT A GLANCE

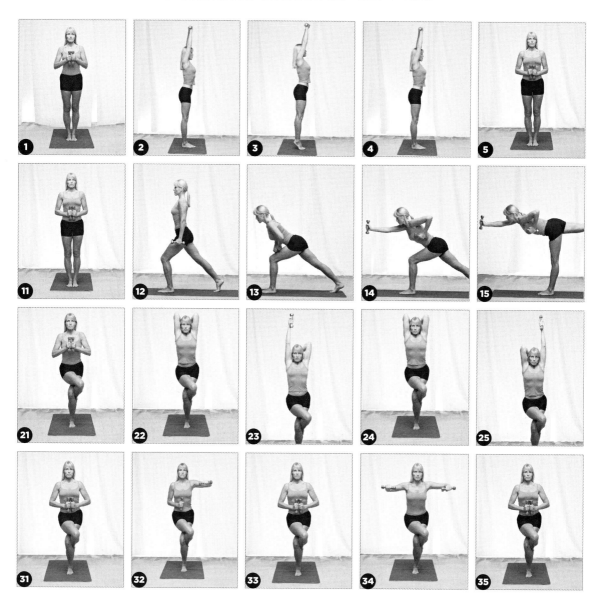

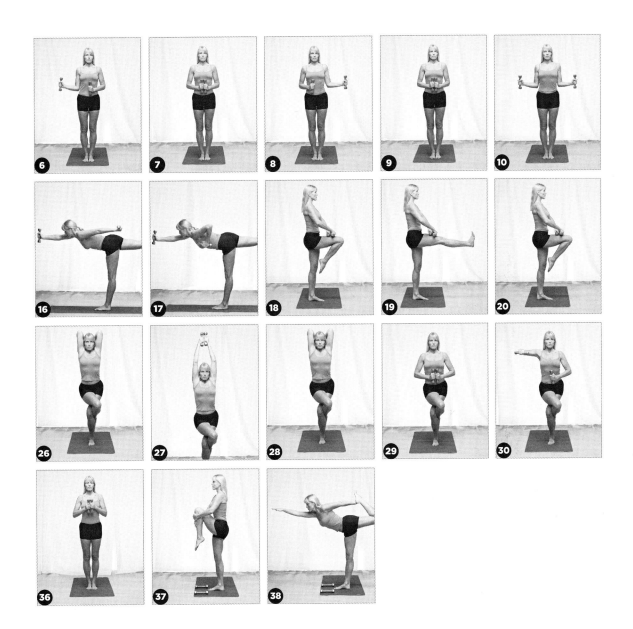

SUN SALUTATION—SEQUENCE 2

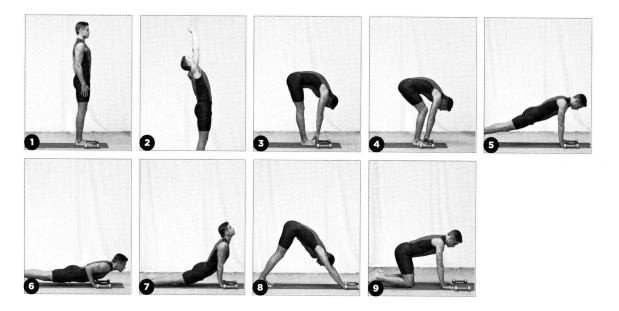

FLOOR POSES
BIRD DOG/FLYING AIRPLANE

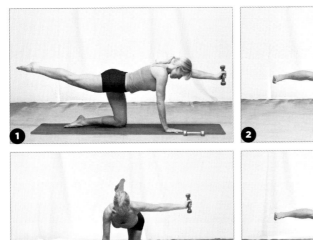

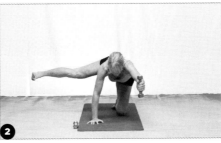

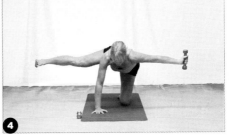

COW/CAT

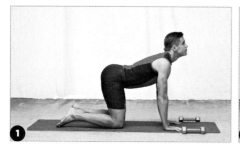 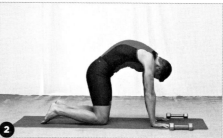

PIGEON

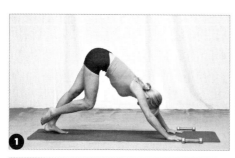 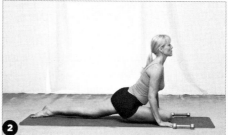

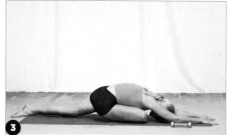 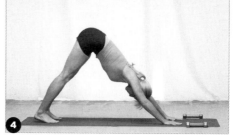

FOREARM PLANK

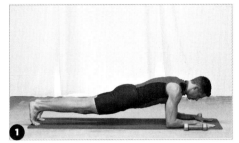

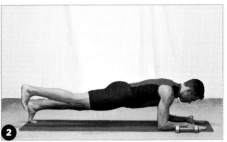

LOCUST

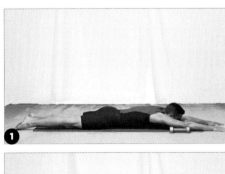

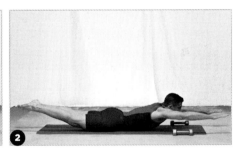

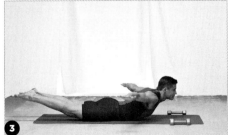

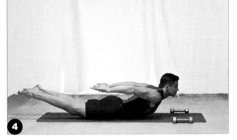

BOW

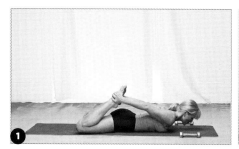 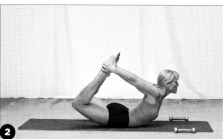

REST

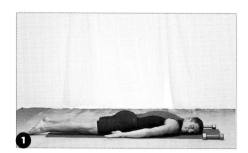

HALF BOAT/FULL BOAT

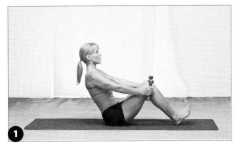

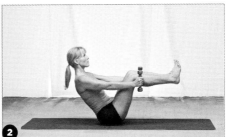

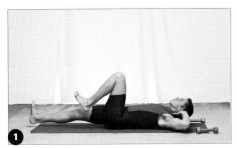

OBLIQUE CRUNCH

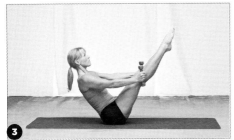

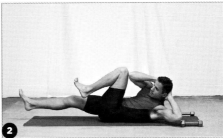

COOLDOWN

RECLINED TWIST

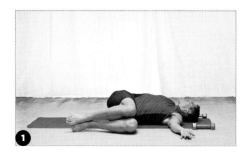

SEATED FORWARD BEND

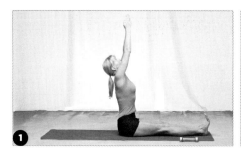
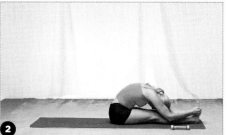

BOUND ANGLE

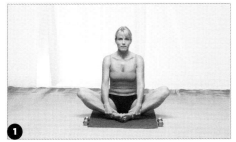 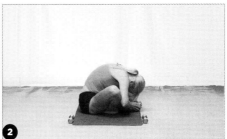

SEATED ONE-LEGGED EXTENSION

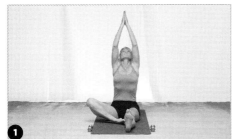 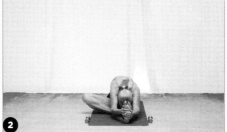

SEATED ONE-LEGGED TWIST

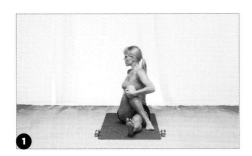

SEATED WIDE-ANGLE SEQUENCE

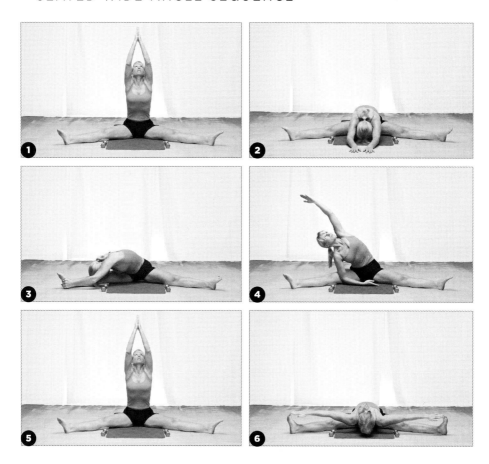

CHILD'S POSE

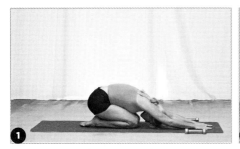

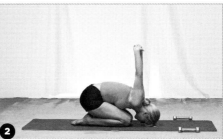

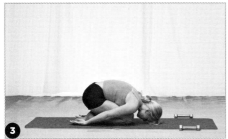

HERO

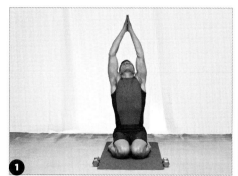 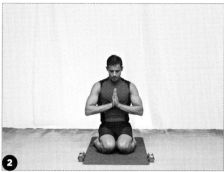

ABOUT THE AUTHORS

Anthony Carillo is a nationally ranked Ironman triathlete and creator of the Iron Yoga® method. He teaches Iron Yoga® classes at several New York City health clubs, and lives with his beautiful wife Amy in New York City. His Web site is www.ironyoga.com

Eric Neuhaus is a writer, journalist, and former television producer for ABC News 20/20. He is also the coauthor of *The World's Fittest You: Four Weeks to Total Fitness*. He lives and works in New York City. Visit him at his Web site at www.ericneuhaus.com.

INDEX

Boldface page references indicate photographs.